Scottish Home and Health Department
Scottish Education Department

Towards Better Health Care for School Children in Scotland

A Report by the Child Health Programme Planning
Group of the Scottish Health Service Planning Council

Edinburgh   Her Majesty's Stationery Office

ISBN 0 11 491648 9

This Report of a Programme Planning Group set up by the Scottish Health Service Planning Council is being published for the information of interested bodies and those concerned with the future planning of health and other relevant services for children.

The Report makes a number of recommendations on various aspects of the service. The Secretary of State will be considering those which require decision by him in the light of the financial resources likely to be available for the health service in Scotland and the recommendations yet to be made by the Scottish Health Service Planning Council on future health priorities.

Foreword

One of the more formidable tasks undertaken by the Child Health Programme Planning Group has been the study of the health care of children while in school, and the improvements which are desirable. It soon became evident that, while the Group was broadly based, in order to make the study really effective the educational and social work representation would have to be strengthened. This was achieved without difficulty and tribute must be paid to the co-opted representatives of those agencies for their diligence and the high quality of their contribution to the work of the Group, and for their generosity in allowing themselves to be treated as full members of the Group.

The study was initiated in three fields—'Surveillance', 'Assessment' and 'Handicap'. There was a fourth—'Dentistry', which is of a slightly different but no less important category and which is the subject of a separate report by the Group. The preliminary study of 'Assessment' and 'Handicap' revealed that the overlap between these two topics was so significant that separate reports were undesirable. In the event, therefore, the Group's study of the school health service proceeded in the two fields which are reflected in the first two sections of this report, namely 'Health Surveillance' and 'Children with Handicap'. As an extension of these studies the Group became involved in questions of staffing and of health records. In this report, therefore, there are included sections dealing with these two important topics.

In addition to the separate report by the Group entitled 'Dental Services for Children at School', to which reference has already been made, the Group has also issued a report entitled 'Vulnerable Families', Whilst the latter report is not directly related to the school health service it cannot be read in isolation. It is important that each of the reports produced by the Group should be read as complementing the others.

It is a matter of convenience that in its reports the Group has made use of a phrase 'the school health service'. This phrase must not be regarded as in any way inhibiting, because the principal objective of the Group has always been and remains to achieve such a measure of integration that there will be a single comprehensive health service for all children from birth until they leave school. The Group has not made a detailed study of the pre-school situation because this has been undertaken by the Paediatric Sub-Committee of the National Medical Consultative Committee. Some system of pre-school developmental screening is a highly desirable prerequisite of the Group's recommendations on health surveillance.

It may be noted that there are substantial similarities between the recommendations made by the Group in the section of its report on 'Children with Handicap' and the proposals put forward in the Warnock report. This is fortuitous because not only has the Group studied this topic from a very different angle from that adopted by the Warnock Committee, but the most radical recommendations contained in this section of the Group's report had already been agreed in principle before the Warnock report became available to the Group.

In its review of 'the school health service' the Group came to appreciate that what it should really be studying is the health care of children. As this study has developed, the importance of the close co-operation between the medical, educational and social work services has become increasingly evident. The section of the Group's report dealing with 'Children with Handicap' emphasises how essential is this close collaboration in order to achieve the continuing comprehensive caring service for children which the Group recognises as its principal aim. The report makes some recommendations regarding the integration and co-ordination of the services provided by these three agencies and favours research into more effective systems of collaboration. This would be expedited by, but must if necessary proceed without, the redistribution of resources.

The Group wishes to thank its sub-committees which did the basic work on the studies dealt with in this report; Dr McArthur and her sub-committee which studied 'Health Surveillance'; Professor Stone and his sub-committee which studied 'Children with Handicap' and Mr Ian Macfadyen and his sub-committee which evaluated the resource implications of the Group's recommendations.

At the conclusion of its deliberations the Group wishes to place on record its appreciation of the invaluable services which it has received from the assessors. Two members of the Secretariat, Mr Robert Mowat, now retired, and Mr W. D.

Wallace have made an outstanding contribution to the work of the Group, which is greatly indebted to both of them.

Richard H. Barclay
Chairman
Child Health Programme Planning Group

November 1979

Child health programme planning group membership

Chairman

Mr R. H. Barclay — Solicitor, Glasgow.

Members

Mr I. Calderwood — Depute Director (Special Education), Grampian Region.

Dr R. K. Ditchburn — General Practitioner, Shetland.

Dr Catherine Frain-Bell — Consultant Paediatrician in Educational Medicine, Tayside Health Board.

Miss J. Himsworth — Health Visitor, Dalkeith Medical Centre.

Miss E. Hocking (resigned 31.3.77) — Principal Social Worker, Royal Hospital for Sick Children, Edinburgh.

Miss O. Hulme — Principal Nursing Officer, Royal Hospital for Sick Children, Glasgow.

Professor J. H. Hutchinson (resigned 1.9.77) — Professor of Child Health, Royal Hospital for Sick Children, Glasgow.

Miss H. Kinloch (appointed 30.6.77) — Senior Social Worker, Royal Aberdeen Children's Hospital.

Dr J. Morag MacArthur — Community Medicine Specialist, Argyll & Clyde Health Board.

Mr A. H. McCall — District Administrator, Perth and Kinross District, Tayside Health Board.

Mr I. J. McDonald — Assistant Principal Psychologist, Child Guidance Service, Strathclyde Region.

Mr I. Macfadyen — Divisional Education Officer, Lothian Region.

Miss C. Milne — Adviser in Early Education, Tayside Regional Council.

Professor R. G. Mitchell (appointed 21.12.77) — Professor of Child Health, University of Dundee.

Dr J. C. Murdoch — General Practitioner and Senior Lecturer, Department of General Practice, University of Dundee.

Miss V. Rennie	Assistant Adviser in Special Education, Strathclyde Region.
Miss P. L. Simon	Area Nursing Officer, Argyll & Clyde Health Board.
Dr A. L. Speirs	Consultant Paediatrician, Stirling Royal Infirmary.
Professor F. H. Stone	Professor of Child and Adolescent Psychiatry, University of Glasgow.
Professor P. Sutcliffe	Professor of Preventive Dentistry, University of Edinburgh.

Assessors

Dr Margaret Bell	Formerly Senior Medical Officer, Scottish Home and Health Department.
Mr D. A. Bennet	Principal, Scottish Home and Health Department.
Dr J. T. Boyd	Senior Medical Officer, Chief Scientist Organisation, Scottish Home and Health Department.
Miss C. L. Boyle	HM Inspector, Inspectorate, Scottish Education Department.
Dr Margaret Hennigan	Senior Medical Officer, Scottish Home and Health Department.
Miss M. H. S. Hunter	Nursing Officer, Scottish Home and Health Department.
Mr J. Urquhart	Principal Research Officer, Information Services Division Common Services Agency.
Miss M. Woodburn	Adviser, Social Work Services Group, Scottish Education Department.

Secretariat

Miss L. R. Maddock (from June, 1978)	Principal, Scottish Health Service Planning Council Secretariat.
Mr R. Mowat (Retired April, 1978)	Principal, Scottish Health Service Planning Council Secretariat
Mr W. D. Wallace	Higher Executive Officer, Scottish Health Service Planning Council Secretariat.

Contents

Appendices

Part I

Health surveillance

Chapter 1   Introduction

1.1 In this part of our report we make proposals for the provision of comprehensive health surveillance for school children.

1.2 Traditionally, the school health service has been organised as a separate entity providing a largely self-contained service. The general extent and content of this service has derived, in the past, from advice issued periodically by the Scottish Home and Health Department to local health authorities, and, since the re-organisation of the Health Service in 1974, to health boards. There is, however, an increasing acceptance of the view that health services in schools should be provided as an integral part of primary health care. There is also a growing emphasis on the need for early identification of disabilities of whatever kind and for close collaboration between the health, educational, social work and other services directed towards children.

1.3 The integration of the primary care services is a theme both of the 'Brotherston' Report by the Sub-Group on Child Health of the Joint Working Party on the Integration of Medical Work[1] and the more recent report of the Court Committee on Child Health Services in England and Wales[2]. These reports emphasise the growing importance of prevention in patterns of care and of the need to bring preventive and curative aspects of care closer together. Chapter 2 of the Brotherston Report sees the objectives of child health services in terms of enabling children to grow and develop as normally as possible, to profit by their education to the full extent of their abilities, and to attain adult life in the best physical, mental and emotional health that can be achieved. In the same vein, the Court Report envisages that the school health service should be concerned with all aspects of a child's health rather than just with the identification and management of particular defects.

1.4 In framing our own proposals we have had regard to the findings of both of these reports on the place of school health in the wider context of health services for children and particularly to the definitions of 'educational medicine' and 'health surveillance' in the Court Report. Our proposals incorporate significant modifications in the present arrangements for examinations of, and specific screening tests for, children at school, and include a number of other suggestions for the operation of the health service within schools. Additionally, we discuss the place of health surveillance in the context of pre-school provision (including nursery schools) in assisting with early identification of problems.

1.5 In Chapter 7 we summarise the resource implications of our proposals. We recognise that there is a lack of data as to the relative effectiveness of the options available. We emphasise the need to monitor and evaluate the various component parts of our suggestions, In particular, we see a need for experimentation and for research projects to study the clinical content of surveillance measures and the effectiveness of delivery of preventive services.

References

[1]*Towards an Integrated Child Health Service*. A report of a joint Working Party on the integration of medical work. Chairman: Sir John Brotherston, Scottish Home and Health Department, Edinburgh, HMSO, 1973.
[2]*Fit for the Future*. The report of the Committee on Child Health Services. Chairman: Professor S. D. M. Court, London, HMSO, 1976. Cmnd. 6684.

Chapter 2   The existing position and the need for change

2.1 The general pattern of school health provision in Scotland was last examined in detail by a Study Group established by the Secretary of State in 1968. This review was followed in 1974 by a report 'The Routine Medical Examination of School Children'[3] produced by a sub-committee of the Consultative Committee of Medical Officers of Health which gives general guidance on the conduct of examinations and draws attention to points of particular importance at certain stages in a child's school career. A separate sub-committee of the Consultative Committee undertook a review[4] of the organisational aspects of school health services in 1974. Taken together, these reports spell out the general framework of guidance at present available to health boards regarding the operation of the health services provided for children in schools.

2.2 Guidance provided by the Scottish Home and Health Department on the pattern of medical examinations and specific screening tests to be incorporated in health surveillance arrangements in schools is contained mainly in Departmental circulars (Reference Nos. NHS 1974 (GEN)77 of 1 November, 1974 and NHS 1975 (GEN)39 of 15 May, 1975). The Department recommended a variation from the previous system of comprehensive medical examinations at each of the three principal stages in a child's school career: only at the school entry stage should a comprehensive examination be undertaken for all children, though the 'leaver' examination (the content of which was not specified) was retained as a further routine procedure. Appendix A shows the coverage of medical examinations of children which was achieved at school entry and school leaving for the year 1977.

2.3 The following is a summary of Departmental guidance in relation to the examinations and tests to be undertaken during a child's school life:

a. *School Entry Stage* (age 5/6 years)
Full medical examination, including hearing and vision tests, carried out on all school entrants.

4

b. *Intermediate Stage* (age 11/12 years)
Universal examinations (formerly carried out at about 9 years) were rejected in favour of a more selective system. Screening tests were retained on a universal basis together with consultation with teachers and school nurses and consideration of parental questionnaires. Medical examinations were to be carried out selectively and timed to have regard to difficulties likely to arise during middle school years.

c. *School Leaver Stage* (age 14/15 years)
After 1972/73 when the school leaving age was raised, the medical examination formerly carried out at age 13/14 was to be carried out at age 14/15. This examination was designed primarily to identify pupils who were unsuitable for certain occupations. Young people staying on at school after age 15 are treated as school leavers.

d. *Separate Screening Tests*
Screening for visual acuity was normally to be carried out every two years in primary school and also at the intermediate and leaver stages. A colour vision test was included at the intermediate stage. Hearing tests by sweep audiometry were suggested at each of the school entry, intermediate and leaver stages.

2.4 The school health service should, in our view, remain the principal provider of health surveillance for all children of school age. Our task has been to seek ways in which it might be possible to achieve greater effectiveness in the detection, treatment and amelioration of significant defects in children. Early detection is a very important factor in achieving this objective and, because of this, our proposals have become involved to some extent in the pre-school stage.

2.5 We agree with the definition of educational medicine given in the Court Report (para. 10.8) and also with the statements made in the Brotherston Report that there is a need for more, not less, expertise and specialisation in educational medicine. Until now much of the work of school doctors has consisted of the identification and supervision of large groups of children with defects of comparatively minor importance. We believe that the time devoted to the routine examination of all school children at certain ages should be reduced in order to free resources which could be deployed to help improve the service for children with particular needs. The recommendations which we make in this report are directed towards this purpose.

References

[3]*The Routine Medical Examination*. Scottish Home and Health Department, Edinburgh, 1973.
[4]*Reorganisation of the School Health Service*. Scottish Home and Health Department, Edinburgh, 1975.

Chapter 3 Recommended programme of medical examinations

3.1 The programme which we recommend for health surveillance at school follows the existing framework of examinations at, or near, the time of school entry, on transfer to secondary school and in the year prior to the school leaving age. We consider that there should be a special examination of individual pupils at any time during school life as and when the need arises (*see* para. 3.27). Our proposals represent the minimum acceptable level of health surveillance. The adequacy of these proposals will need to be monitored and evaluated over a period of time.

Pre-school developmental screening

3.2 In our view the maximum benefit to the child will be achieved if the health surveillance programme in schools is linked to a comprehensive system of pre-school developmental screening. We have examined the developmental screening protocol* proposed by the Paediatric Sub-Committee of the National Medical Consultative Committee and we agree that a system on similar lines should be brought into use to cover all children.

3.3 We wish to emphasise the importance of early notification to education and social work authorities of children with significant abnormalities, so that these authorities may take whatever steps are appropriate in the circumstances. In the case of education authorities this will include planning the educational services which the handicapped child is going to require and arranging for any intervention at the pre-school stage which may help parents with their child's early education. In the case of social work departments this will assist them in arranging to provide continuing support for, and practical assistance to, families with handicapped children. The aim should be that, wherever possible, any disability which has an educational implication should be notified by age three. In cases of severe handicap, notification should be made at the earliest possible time. By notification we do not imply any formal procedure but simply the communication of a child's need to the appropriate authority.

---

*This 'Developmental Screening Protocol' is an unpublished document prepared by the Paediatric Sub-Committee in 1977.

6

Nursery schools, playgroups and day nurseries

3.4 Although we have stressed the importance which we attach to the developmental screening of pre-school children, we recognise that total coverage may be difficult to achieve in the short term. For this reason we have considered whether some of the resources at present devoted to the school health service should be redeployed with a view to improving the health surveillance coverage of the pre-school population. In particular, we have considered whether the experience gained in carrying out health surveillance in schools should be applied to identifiable groups of pre-school children. Some children attending nursery schools are already included in the school health surveillance programme, but this is not so in the case of children attending playgroups or day nurseries. We recommend that, until a universal developmental screening programme can be implemented, special arrangements should be made to carry out health surveillance of those groups of children identifiable by attendance at nursery schools, playgroups and day nurseries. Wherever possible, at least one parent should be present when the child is seen, both for reassurance and particularly to enable the maximum amount of information about the child's emotional background and development to be obtained.

3.5 For all such children records should be examined by a member of the school health team to ensure that the child's developmental screening is up to date. Where it is not, or where records are unavailable or incomplete, the appropriate developmental screening examinations should be carried out as soon as possible after parental consent has been obtained. Because of the restricted number of children in some playgroups and the absence of appropriate facilities in the premises in which many of them are held, special arrangements for the examinations may have to be made. In costing this recommendation we have tried to make some allowance for the logistical problems involved, which we recognise may not be inconsiderable.

3.6 As pre-school developmental screening programmes become established, an increasing proportion of children attending nursery schools, playgroups and day nurseries may no longer require medical examination under school health service arrangements. Nevertheless there will be a continuing need for health surveillance in these establishments. We therefore recommend that nurses should carry out an annual review of all children in nursery schools and that doctors should visit on a regular basis. Wherever possible similar arrangements should be made for playgroups and day nurseries.

3.7 We do not wish to identify specifically the staff who would provide health surveillance in these situations because this question is only one aspect of the much wider problem of integrating the method of delivery of health care to pre-school children and to school children. This problem does not fall entirely within the remit of our Group or within the context of this report.

During first school year

3.8 We consider that all children should continue to have a comprehensive examination during the first year in school. We have considered the arguments in favour of carrying out this examination before or after school entry. Attendance at school provides the first occasion when those operating a health surveillance programme can be sure of access to virtually every child. It is our view that, provided there are adequate pre-school developmental screening arrangements in operation, there are considerable advantages to be obtained by waiting until children are attending primary school. It is essential that where pre-school developmental screening has been carried out, the child's records should be made available at the time of school entry together with any additional relevant health data including details of any regular medication prescribed. The child's general practitioner should be informed when this or any other examination is to take place, and invited to supply any relevant information in his possession. Before the medical examination is carried out, a questionnaire should be sent to parents for completion (see para. 5.5). We recommend that particular attention should be paid to children whose parents do not return the questionnaire or who fail to complete it adequately.

3.9 Where there is no evidence that adequate pre-school developmental screening has been carried out, the school entry medical examination should be undertaken as early in the child's school life as practicable. For other children there are advantages in delaying the school entry examination until the teacher has had an opportunity to form an impression of the child's physical, emotional and intellectual development.

Before transfer to secondary school

3.10 We have considered the arguments for and against having a routine medical review of all children at the time of transfer to secondary school. We feel that there is a need for a formal medical review between school entry and school leaving. We believe that such a review would lessen the possibility of developments during the pupil's early years in school being overlooked, especially those with potential vocational and consequent educational implications.

3.11 We recommend that a formal review of all children's medical records should be undertaken during the child's last year at primary school. It is probable that at this time children will still be under the supervision of one particular teacher whose comments would be of special value when selecting those for medical examination. Teachers of physical education should also be asked for comments. As in the case of the school entry examination, the review of records should be supplemented by a questionnaire to be completed by parents (*see* para. 5.5) and the pupil's general practitioner should be informed of the review and invited to provide any relevant information which may be in his possession.

3.12 On the basis of this review, children will be selected for medical examination. It can be particularly difficult to identify those children likely to have an emotional or psychiatric disorder and evidence from the observant parent or teacher can be most helpful. Behavioural changes such as unusual solitariness, inattention and drowsiness, physical complaints including changes in weight or appetite, vomiting, recurring pains or alteration of toilet habit would suggest the need for medical examination. In the child's personal history, recent hospital admission, current medical supervision, regular medication, prolonged or frequent absences from school, with or without parental knowledge, and learning or behavioural problems sufficient to have warranted referral to the child guidance service would all suggest that the child should be examined. Particular attention should also be paid to those pupils known to be living in disadvantageous circumstances. We recommend that children in respect of whom parental questionnaires are not adequately completed should be specially considered for examination.

3.13 Our recommendations for the school transfer examination are unlikely to have additional resource implications. We consider, however, that it is important that the process of selection should be placed on a more systematic basis than is the case at present, not least because there is a need to assess the extent to which the selective examination fails to detect significant health problems. Evidence on this point is limited and conflicting. We recommend that a national research exercise should be mounted to validate the use of selection by examining a control group of children. The design of a major project of this kind is outwith the scope of this Group, but it would clearly have very important implications for record design and for the standardised definition and recording of those child health-related problems agreed to be of significance.

Before leaving school

3.14 In the school year before that in which the pupil reaches the statutory leaving age his medical record should be reviewed together with questionnaires returned by parents (*see* para. 5.5). In the light of this review and, where appropriate, after consultation with parents, teachers, careers officers, general practitioners and other professionals, arrangements should be made to examine all children who may seem to have a disability with vocational implications. All children identified at the earlier transfer to secondary school review as having a problem should be examined, as should any child in respect of whom a problem has come to notice during secondary school. In addition, in the absence of any other indication, an examination should be carried out in any case if the pupil or the parents express a wish for it.

3.15 A review at this stage should identify children with disabilities which should be reported in due course to the Employment Medical Advisory Service, children with disabilities which are not significant in terms of choice of employment but who will require continuing attention from the health or other services during the remaining period of schooling and possibly thereafter, and the presence of adverse social or psychological factors which may affect the child's health.

3.16 When the school doctor considers that a child has some medical, physical or mental impairment which could impose difficulty or danger in certain occupations, form Y9 is completed and copies sent to the employment medical adviser, careers officer and family doctor. We are conscious that selective examinations at school leaving stage involve a risk of failure to identify some children who have health problems with vocational implications. We attach considerable importance to the validation, by the examination of control groups, of the use of selection (*see* para. 3.13).

3.17 The benefit of introducing a selective examination prior to school leaving will be to reduce considerably the number of medical examinations carried out at present in many areas. This will release some medical staff resources which could be redeployed elsewhere. There is evidence that in some areas it has not proved possible to comply with present Departmental advice, and clearly in those areas no resource saving can be expected from the use of selection (*see* Chapter 7) Nursing staff resources are unlikely to be affected by the recommendation.

Supplementary routine examinations

3.18 In addition to these principal medical examinations there is need for supplementary routine examinations for special purposes.

Height and weight

3.19 Height and weight measurements should be taken annually for all children in primary school, and also for secondary pupils but on a selective basis. This should be done by the school nurse using equipment which is capable of giving acceptably accurate results. The results should be recorded on percentile charts, such as Tanner's charts, in order to facilitate immediate recognition of any deviation from normal development. Periodically, equipment should be checked for accuracy.

Health care interview

3.20 A personal interview with each pupil by the school nurse should be held annually to help the nurse and the pupil to get to know each other and to encourage discussion on general health matters or specific problems then or later. The opportunity should be taken to explain to the pupils the ways in which advice may be obtained. It might be convenient to try to arrange this interview to coincide with the annual check on height and weight. We think that on average 10 minutes per pupil should be allowed for this interview. This recommendation has substantial implications for nurse staffing and training.

Vision

3.21 We have considered papers provided by the National Optical Consultative Committee and the Orthoptic Sub-Committee of the National Para-Medical Consultative Committee. These papers proposed that visual screening of pre-school children should be carried out by orthoptists and that such screening should be done at an early age (1 year–18 months approximately) to detect congenital defects and early onset of squint, and at a later age when a subjective visual acuity test can be carried out ($3\frac{1}{2}$ years–4 years) to detect the later onset of squint. Early identification of defects such as strabismus would ensure that remedial action could be taken before school entry and at a time when treatment would be most effective. In our view there may therefore be an advantage in bringing forward the visual acuity test to be associated with the pre-school health surveillance programme at age 3. We have considered the proposal that this screening programme for visual defects should be carried out by orthoptists. On the evidence presented we are not satisfied, that screening by orthoptists is necessary nor are we convinced that such a scheme would represent an efficient use of resources in present circumstances. In addition, we believe that the difficulty of achieving full coverage of the pre-school child population in a special vision screening programme may have been under-estimated. We recommend that vision screening in the pre-school years should, for the time being, be carried out by doctors or health visitors in the course of routine developmental screening examinations or in the course of visits to children in their homes. When screening for visual defects has been carried out, all cases of suspected squint and all of the cases where any measure of doubt remains should be referred for orthoptic examination in the first instance. This proposal would restrict the very heavy calls upon orthoptic and administrative resources, which the National Optical Consultative Committee programme would involve, and would also reduce the time spent by ophthalmologists in examining children who do not have visual defects, thus meeting one of the principal objectives of their orthoptic screening programme. In making this recommendation, we realise that neither proposal has been properly validated in terms of effectiveness and cost. We recommend that studies should be undertaken to compare the relative cost-effectiveness of visual screening of the pre-school children carried out by orthoptists with screening carried out by doctors and health visitors during the course of their routine contacts with children.

3.22 We have received advice from a number of sources on the timing of tests for visual acuity during school life. The advice has been contradictory. We recommend that testing should be carried out at school entry, at ages 7–8, 11 and 14/15 years (secondary school leaving age). We do not consider that there is any compelling medical reason for selecting these ages in preference to others, but we believe that they fit reasonably into the educational and vocational guidance framework.

3.23 The test at 11 years should include examination for colour vision defects carried out by the nurse. Earlier examination is of doubtful reliability and cannot be recommended. In this connection we commend the National Optical Consultative Committee's proposal that education authorities should be asked to discuss the possibility of discontinuing the use in teaching of colours likely to cause difficulty to those who are colour defective. When the presence of a colour defect seems to conflict with a preference for a particular career, a detailed colour vision examination should be made.

Hearing

3.24 We agree with the Advisory Committee on Services for Hearing Impaired People that an adequate system of screening for hearing defects is an essential component of the pre-school developmental programme. We recommend, as did the Committee, that screening for hearing defects by sweep audiometry should be carried out at school entry and again at age 8 years. We are aware that hearing screening is at present carried out by a variety of staff, usually school nurses or health visitors or audiometricians. We are more concerned that this test should be undertaken completely by suitably trained staff than that it should be carried out by any particular person. We are interested to note that the ACSHIP report recommends that a school nurse with suitable training is the appropriate person to carry out screening for hearing defects. We agree with this recommendation, provided that it is understood that such screening is part of the nurse's total role. We recognise nevertheless, that existing staffing patterns would render this arrangement impracticable or inappropriate in some areas, in the short term. Audiometricians are employed to undertake this work in a number of health board areas and in such cases we would not wish to suggest any change.

Cleanliness and infestation

3.25 It is our belief that examination for cleanliness or infestation should be a part of health surveillance and not normally a task carried out in isolation. It is a degrading process which may adversely affect the child's relationship with the health team. In areas where there is persistent lack of cleanliness or infestation prevails there may be need for regular examinations. We consider that this type of examination does not require the training and expertise of a qualified nurse and that it could be carried out by a nursing auxiliary, or other aide with appropriate training, in consultation with a qualified nurse. We do not see it as a routine function of the School Health Service to disinfest children but to educate parents and children if old enough to do this themselves. There is still a continuing need for the present legal powers to ensure that where persuasion fails, after notification, a child is cleaned or disinfested.

Foot defects

3.26 We have received advice from the Chiropody Sub-Committee of the National Para-Medical Consultative Committee whose main proposal is that chiropodists should be employed in the school health service for the detection of actual and potential foot defects by universal examination of children at the age of 9 years. We are inclined to doubt the feasibility of this proposal as a universal proposition in existing circumstances. Examples of the extent of defects among school children provided by the Chiropody Sub-Committee seem to indicate that the training of school nurses should be more closely orientated towards the examination of feet. We recommend that the occasion of the annual interview by the school nurse should be used for inspection of feet followed, if necessary, by further referral.

Special measures

3.27 We have already recommended that a special examination should be undertaken whenever required. The need for this might be identified as a result of information received from doctor, nurse, teacher, educational psychologist, social worker, parent or pupil. In addition, we believe that, unless contraindicated, when a child has had a prolonged absence (ie a period of over 4 weeks) or frequent short absences from school whether for medical or other reasons, consideration should be given, as a matter of routine, to the desirability of a call from the health visitor followed up, if necessary, by a special medical examination. Prolonged or frequent absence from school must, itself, impose an educational handicap and we think it important that any contributory or complicating medical factor should be properly assessed.

Content of Medical Examinations

3.28 Existing guidance on the content of school medical examinations has been considered at our request by the Paediatric Sub-Committee of the National Medical Consultative Committee. With the Sub-Committee's comments in mind, we recommend that, in programming sessions, a minimum of 20 minutes per pupil should be allocated in the case of the three principal school medical examinations exclusive of the time required for documentation.

Summary

3.29 We have summarised our health surveillance programme for children at school on page 15.

Summary of health surveillance programme for children at school

Location	Approx. Age	Review Records	Universal Medical Examination	Selective Medical Examination	Special Medical Examination	Visual Acuity	Colour Vision	Sweep Audiometry	Annual Interview with nurse	Height and Weight Measurement	Foot Inspection	Cleanliness Inspection
Primary School	4-6	+	+		*+	+		+	+	+	+	+
	6-7				+			+	+	+	+	+
	7-8				*+				+	+	+	+
	8-9				+	+			+	+	+	+
	9-10	+			*+				+	+	+	+
	10-11			+	+				+	+	+	+
Secondary School	11-12				*+	+	+		+	*+	+	+
	12-13				+				+	*+	+	+
	13-14	+			*+				+	*+	+	+
	14-15			+	+	+			+	*+	+	+
	15-16				*+				+	*+	+	+

*As indicated.

15

Chapter 4   Coverage of child population and application to special groups

4.1 In our view, a system of health surveillance should extend to all children. We are concerned, therefore, to ensure that there are no groups of children who do not receive the benefits of a health surveillance programme.

Extension to List D schools and grant-aided and independent schools for the handicapped

4.2 At present children receiving certain types of education do not automatically come under the care of the school health service. Included in this category are children at List D schools—although we are aware that the future of these schools is currently under discussion—grant-aided residential special schools and independent day schools for the handicapped. We consider that, since the children who are attending such schools are in many cases the responsibility of education authorities and dependent on the provision of intensive health and other caring services, it would be logical for the school health service to be extended to include them. The numbers are relatively small. Although the health surveillance programme which we recommend could be applied to some handicapped children only in modified forms we regard it as important that the general health of such children should come under regular review. It is desirable to arrange for grant-aided and independent day schools for the handicapped to benefit from the same health service as education authority day schools in the area. We therefore recommend that the health surveillance programme be extended to include children attending List D Schools and grant-aided and independent day schools for handicapped children. In making this recommendation we are aware that there are complicating factors. In the first place, since the local health board does not have an absolute duty to extend the school health service to such schools, any provision would need to be a matter for agreement. Secondly, under existing legislation there could be no absolute assurance that the programme offered to a private school (whether a day or boarding school) would reach each child, since the power of the education authority to require the parent to present the child for examination would be lacking. Legislation may be necessary to achieve this.

4.3 It is not possible within the compass of this report to suggest how a health surveillance programme covering the years of schooling could be devised for these special groups, or how the programme should be delivered in each case. Once, however, a basic programme is established we think that it would be for experts in the field of individual handicaps to devise appropriate programmes for their own groups. In the residential situation there may be opportunity to combine the general practitioner services and continuing health surveillance in one appointment.

Extension to other grant-aided and independent schools

4.4 We regard the provision of the school health service to other grant-aided and independent schools as being intrinsically desirable and we recommend that it should be undertaken by or under the supervision of health boards. We appreciate that this would have resource implications for boards, but because of the uneven geographic distribution of such schools and the uncertainty of the uptake of the service, which could be variable, we have not attempted meantime to quantify or cost these implications.

Follow-up of non-attending children

4.5 We emphasise the importance of a positive follow-up of children who do not attend routine sessions of any part of the health surveillance programme. Initially this should be done by arranging further appointments but, should this fail, the child should, if necessary, be visited at home. We see the health visitor as having a crucial role to play in this follow-up process and we strongly endorse recommendations which have been made elsewhere on the paramount importance of adequate levels of health visitor staffing, particularly in areas where there is known to be a high incidence of social, educational and health problems. We would prefer to see this follow-up implemented by persuasion, but we recognise that there will be occasions where persuasion will fail and where the interests of the child will make it essential for a new legal power to be made available so that the existing power to fine the parents of a defaulting child is extended to authorise the medical examination of a child in the absence of its parents' consent. The method of enforcement requires further thought, having regard to existing diffuse legislation relating to the well-being of children, and, as such, is outwith the scope of this report.

4.6 We are aware that the type of follow-up proposal which we advocate is bound to be relatively expensive in its use of staff resources and that the effectiveness of those proposals has not been adequately validated. We therefore recommend that consideration be given to mounting a study to assess the cost-effectiveness of such a proposal.

Other measures

4.7 We have considered other measures which might be taken in order to attain full coverage of the child population by the health surveillance programme. We consider that there is a need to examine means by which any change of address could be more effectively communicated amongst the various agencies involved in health, education and social work. We recommend in agreement with the Court Committee that, on claiming child benefit, there should be a requirement to notify any change of address.

4.8 It has been suggested that compliance with the recommended developmental screening and health surveillance programme for children should be reinforced by making it a pre-requisite for receiving child benefit. At first sight this is an attractive incentive which could be expected to have an immediate and obvious effect on the motivation of most parents. However, it has not yet been proved to be effective and, further, this sanction could impose a financial disadvantage on some families who are in need. We cannot support the implementation of this proposal.

Chapter 5 Involvement of parents and older children

5.1 We are convinced that the involvement of parents should be an integral part of the conduct of health surveillance programmes. It is important that they should receive letters and questionnaires well in advance of examinations or reviews. Health boards in conjunction with education authorities will have to decide how this can best be achieved.

5.2 The school doctor should write to parents simply phrased letters explaining clearly the purpose and nature of any forthcoming examination.

5.3 Individual health boards will have their own views on the terms of such letters, but we think the following points might, with advantage, be included in letters sent out prior to the school entry examination:

a. an explanation of the general purpose of the health surveillance programme and an outline of its content;

b. a reference to the examination/screening in prospect, its likely timing and the desirability of parental attendance;

c. an explanation of the purpose of the questionnaire and an assurance of confidentiality in the use of information given;

d. confirmation that the general practitioner has been informed about, and consulted about, the forthcoming examination;

e. an undertaking to communicate to the parents any significant outcome of the examination/screening test.

5.4 We recognise that it is the education authority rather than the health board which has the statutory power to require the parent to present the child for examination. The letter should, therefore, make clear that, in inviting the parent to present the child for examination, the doctor is acting as an agent of the education authority.

5.5 We have already referred to the use of questionnaires to parents to elicit information relevant to medical examinations or reviews. A carefully phrased questionnaire if completed and returned by the parent can be of considerable assistance to the school doctor in providing a comprehensive picture. We do not make a recommendation as to the detailed design of the questionnaire, but Appendix B shows the type of data which it might be appropriate to collect by this means.

5.6 We consider it important that all parents and older children should have access to the health team responsible for a school and that they should be made aware of the facilities in existence and how they can make use of them. The recommended introduction of the health interview with the school nurse should help to meet this need. The school nurse will be responsible where appropriate for referring the child to other members of the health team.

5.7 We are aware of the importance which is placed by some bodies on the availability of self referral 'clinics'. While we agree with the principle of the free availability of confidential advice, we are conscious of the need to ensure that the resource implications of the recommendations which we make lie within the bounds of practicality. We do not consider that it would be productive to commit a large proportion of doctors' time to staffing 'walk-in' clinics save in exceptional circumstances. We recommend that access to advice for parents or pupils should normally be through the school nurse who will regularly be present in the school, and who will be known to the teaching staff and pupils. It should be the responsibility of the school nurse to refer the case, as appropriate, to other members of the health team, or to a worker in another discipline. Although we consider that the normal approach should be through the school nurse, there will be occasions when it will be necessary for there to be direct access by the parent or pupil to the school doctor. Provision should be made to ensure that this is possible and that the means of contacting the school doctor is known to parents and pupils.

5.8 Any arrangement for access by parents and pupils to the school doctor should have proper regard for the relationship of parents and pupils with their general practitioner. Discussion between parents and the school doctor should normally pertain to matters concerning the health of the child in school or arising out of an examination or a screening test carried out on the child by the school health team. If matters arise which are clearly more appropriate to the general practitioner they should naturally be referred to him in the usual way.

Chapter 6   The interchange of information between school health and other professional staff

6.1 If any system of health surveillance is to be effective those responsible for its operation must have access to all relevant information subject to any constraints imposed by its confidential nature. The availability of information will depend to a large extent on good communications between, on the one side, the school doctor and nurse and, on the other side, the teacher, the educational psychologist, those working in primary medical care and medical specialist services and the social worker. In this part of our report we have concerned ourselves with the question of working relationships only in so far as they are relevant to the suggested programme of examinations. Matters relating to the involvement of school health staff with other professionals in the assessment and management of handicapped children are discussed in Part II of this report.

Relationship with teachers

6.2 Teachers are in a particularly good position to notice changes in a child's pattern of behaviour and to detect deviations from normal performance. Being in contact with the child regularly, and in some cases for an extensive period during each school day, the teacher may be the person best placed, apart from the child's parents, to notice an actual or potential health problem.

6.3 If a free and useful exchange of information between the school health team and teachers is to be achieved, it is essential that there should be an adequate health presence in the school. We recommend that each school should have a named school doctor, nurse and health visitor and that each should visit the school sufficiently frequently to become personally known to the staff.

6.4 We consider that in a large secondary school the nurse's duties would require her to be present for some part of each day. In certain schools in areas of multiple deprivation there may be a need for a nurse to be present all day. This would afford ample opportunity for her to become the known point of contact between the teaching staff, the pupils, and the health services. The position is more difficult in some of the smaller schools, particularly in primary schools, where the volume of work which the nurse has to do might not, of itself, necessitate her frequent attendance. Despite this, we consider that it is essential that a credible health presence be maintained in every school and we recommend that the school nurse should visit all schools for which she has responsibility not less frequently than once a week. We do not consider that a name and a telephone number to be called in case of need, although essential in itself, is an adequate substitute for regular meetings and discussions, formal and informal, between the nurse and members of the teaching staff.

6.5 It is the practice in some schools for all contacts with the school doctor to be made through the head teacher. While we appreciate the need for head teachers to be kept informed, we consider that it is very important that the school doctor should be known to all members of the teaching staff and we believe that any teacher should be able to make informal contact directly with the school doctor. If all requests for medical advice have to be channelled officially through the head teacher this must militate against ready communication because the tendency will be for the teacher to refer problems to the school doctor only when they have reached major proportions. We accept nevertheless that the head teacher must be the official point of contact for the formal requests for information which precede medical examinations or reviews.

Relationship with general practitioners

6.6 General practitioners have a most important role to play in the school health service, whether by acting as school doctors, or, if that is not possible, by working closely in conjunction with those carrying out this function. It is essential that there should be a free exchange of all relevant information between general practitioners and school doctors where these are not the same person. Each should be able to refer to, or consult with, the other without difficulty and without undue formality. School doctors need to be aware of important episodes of ill health, and reports of hospital consultations and investigations should be made available to them as a matter of routine. It is also important that general practitioners should be informed of significant findings resulting from medical examinations and screening tests carried out by the school health service.

Relationship with community nurses

6.7 In the past the school nurse has tended to work in isolation from her nursing colleagues in primary care. There would be a real benefit if she were more closely associated with the primary care team. This could be achieved either through health visitor links with the school or by involving the school nurse in a direct association with a particular primary care team. This would be a more realistic proposition in cases where the school catchment and general practice areas have similar boundaries.

Other relationships

6.8 The health surveillance programme which we have recommended will bring the school doctor and nurse into contact with dental officers[5] and para-medical staff. We recommend that this should be a recognised procedure for ensuring that the findings of para-medical personnel involved in screening examinations are brought to the attention of the appropriate medical and educational staff. The responsibility for establishing and carrying out the procedure should rest with the school doctor and nurse.

6.9 School health staff, in carrying out health surveillance, must have regular contact with colleagues working in the child guidance, child and adolescent psychiatric and social work services. These professionals should be known to each other so that easy lines of communication on matters relating to the welfare of school children can be established.

6.10 Where a child has been referred to an educational psychologist and/or a child psychiatrist we recommend that the school doctor should be kept informed of his progress and of any measures which have been taken to ameliorate the situation.

Records

6.11 We have already made some reference to records and this subject is dealt with more fully in Part IV of this report. There is one recurrent difficulty which is of great concern and which merits an immediate statement. It has been repeatedly brought to our notice that there is no standardised procedure for the transfer of school medical records between schools in different geographical areas. This results in records being sent to a variety of destinations—schools, general practitioners and records officers amongst others. Under these circumstances, not only do records go missing but also it is almost impossible to maintain a proper level of confidentiality. Prior to reorganisation of the Health Service, the Medical Officer of Health was the nominated doctor to whom records and information should be forwarded. It is our belief that a clearly identified doctor holding the same post in all health boards should have responsibility for requesting and receiving school health records from outwith the area. We therefore recommend that the Community Medicine Specialist with responsibility for child health should be responsible for this task.

References

[5] *Dental Services for Children at School*. A report of the Child Health Programme Planning Group of the Scottish Health Service Planning Council. Chairman: Professor Philip Sutcliffe, Scottish Home and Health Department, Edinburgh, HMSO, 1980. Paragraphs 4.15–4.21.

Chapter 7 Resource implications

METHOD OF WORKING

7.1 We listed the broad aims of the school health service as a series of functions. We then redefined them as objectives and the activities required to achieve them. For each objective, activities were further refined into a flow chart in which all the necessary steps required to perform the activity were placed in logical sequence and the interrelations between them indicated. From the flow chart a corresponding detailed worksheet was derived on which the activities were listed in sequence. The type of staff best suited to perform each activity was then agreed although no attempt was made to distinguish between categories of medical or nursing staff. We have set these out at Appendix C. We did not quantify the effect of the recommendations on the levels of non-nursing and non-medical staff as we were agreed that any changes would be entirely consequential on changes in the professional staff complement.

7.2 It should be noted that, in making estimates of the staff implications of the recommendation to make special arrangements for health surveillance of playgroup children, the assumption has been made that these medical services will be provided by the school health service. This assumption has been used only as a method of arriving at an estimate of staff resources required to implement our recommendations, on the basis that the overall resource implications will be similar irrespective of the organisational structure or type of staff providing services. It must not be inferred that we recommend that these services should be provided exclusively by the school health service. (*See* para. 3.7.)

7.3 We came to the conclusion that of our recommendations three, which involve a change from the status quo within the school health service, would have considerable resource implications. These recommendations are:

(a) Special arrangements for the health surveillance of children attending playgroups and day nurseries.

(b) Selective examination at school leaving.

(c) Nurse-pupil interviews.

24

In addition, the recommendation to extend the school health service to all independent schools (*see* para. 4.4) may have substantial resource implications, but we did not cost these because of the uneven geographic distribution of such schools and uncertainty about the extent of uptake of the service.

7.4 Quantification was hampered by the paucity of relevant information relating to the school health service. National statistics relating to school health examinations are restricted to:

(a) the number of school health examinations at school entry and school leaving.

(b) the number of defects found at these examinations.

At the same time routine staffing statistics relate only to

(c) the number of whole time equivalent clinical medical officers and senior clinical officers in post.

Clearly these data alone are inadequate to permit quantification of changes affecting specific components of the school health service. For this reason members of our Group were asked to provide estimates, from their own health boards, of the medical staff resources required to carry out each activity (or group of activities) identified on the work sheets. These estimates were compared where possible with data provided by community medicine specialists (child health) for several health boards.

7.5 We then calculated the proportion of time spent on the following for one health board for which a complete set of data was available:

(a) nursery school children examinations;

(b) school entry examinations;

(c) examinations at school transfer (or, as at present in some health boards, at another date);

(d) school leaving examinations;

(e) special examinations and examinations in special schools;

(f) administration;

and for nurses

(g) annual primary school examinations;

(h) vaccination and immunisation;

(i) other nursing activities.

From these base line figures it is possible to express both the present staff resources allocated to activities and any increase in staff resources resulting from any of our recommendations as a proportion of existing staff resources. Estimates provided by members of our Group are considered to be 'best estimates' within the constraints imposed upon us.

7.6 Additional information was required relating to the following (figures in parentheses are estimates made by us):
  (a) The proportion of children which would be examined if a selective examination were introduced (25%).
  (b) The size of control group required to monitor the selective examination (5%).
  (c) The number of children who would refer themselves if a selective examination were introduced at school leaving age (30%).
  (d) The allowance that should be made for travel to playgroups and day nurseries to carry out medical examinations (50% of time spent examining children).

Estimates for items (a) and (b) were based on suitable extrapolations from
  (i) Information from the Isle of Wight study which relates to children aged 10–12.
  (ii) Information from health districts in Scotland in which selection is already practised at age 11.

7.7 The method of calculation also took into account changes in the school age population as projected by the Registrar General for 1981, 1986 and 1991. Projections based on 1973, 1974 and 1975 populations are available and because of the differing assumptions used in each of these, considerable difference exists between them in the expected size of the 1991 population. For this reason we felt that population projections did not provide a reliable basis for estimating changes in demands placed on the school health service beyond 1986. However, it may be anticipated that a decline of up to 12% may occur in the school population by 1986. Appendix D shows projections of numbers of children aged 5, 11 and 16 years in 1981, 1986 and 1991.

7.8 Clearly, objections can be raised to the methods of working which we adopted. These fall into two categories:
  (a) Objections that the magnitude of error in the estimates may be such as to invalidate the method.
  (b) Objections that the extrapolation from the experience of health boards to provide national estimates is not justified.

We have considered both types of objection in order to establish whether we should advise that quantification of our recommendations was not possible. We felt, however, that the estimates do provide a useful basis for quantifying the resource implications of our recommendations, provided an appropriate caveat is accepted, ie that the derived figures provide a yard stick for estimating the scale rather than the absolute magnitude of the cost of implementing our recommendations.

RESULTS OF THE QUANTIFICATION EXERCISE

7.9 In estimating the magnitude of the change in staff resources required to meet our recommendations, we made the assumption that at present all health boards have adequate resources to comply with existing national advice. Where, however, this is not the case additional resources will be required.

Medical staff implications of recommendations

7.10 The results of our quantification in respect of medical staff are summarised in Table 1. The potential savings in medical staff resources resulting from population change are also shown for the purposes of comparison. We have estimated that the introduction of selection in the school leaving examination will save about 5% of the existing medical staff resources allocated to the school health service. The extension of medical examinations to playgroups and day nurseries will require an increase of about 15% of existing medical staff resources assuming that all nursery school children at present receive a medical examination.

Nursing staff implications of recommendations

7.11 Table 2 summarises the results of our quantification in respect of nursing staff. The potential savings in nursing staff resources resulting from population change are also shown for purposes of comparison. It can be seen that the introduction of a selective examination at school leaving does not appear likely to have any significant effect on the amount of nursing staff resources required to carry out this examination. The increase in the resources required to provide nursing staff for examinations for play school and day nursery children is proportionately the same as for medical staff but amounts to 6% of existing school nurse resources as opposed to 15% in the case of doctors.

7.12 Additional resources will also be required to meet the recommendation for a nurse to interview each pupil at each age for which a full medical examination is not conducted. The overall effect of this recommendation is an increase of 6% of existing nursing staff resources. The net effect of the recommendations is thus to increase the nursing staff resources required by some 12%.

Table 1 Medical staff costs of recommendations expressed as % of existing medical staff resources allocated to school health service

Cost of making special arrangements for health surveillance of children at play-groups and day nurseries	+15%
Cost of introducing selective examination	− 5%
TOTAL cost of recommendations as % of existing medical staff resources	+10%
Potential effect on costs of population changes—1981	− 7%
—1986	−10%
—1991	*
Cost of Abandoning Selection at Age 11[1] as % of existing medical staff resources	+ 8%

*Figure not reliable for purposes of this exercise.
[1]Not one of our recommendations, but included for comparison purposes.

Table 2 Nursing staff costs of recommendations expressed as % of existing nursing staff resources allocated to school health service

Cost of making special arrangements for health surveillance of children at play-groups and day nurseries	+ 6%
Cost of introducing selective examination at school leaving	0%
Cost of introducing nurse pupil interviews	+ 6%
TOTAL cost of recommendations as % of existing medical staff resources	+12%
Potential effect on costs of population change—1981	− 7%
—1986	−10%
—1991	*
Cost of Abandoning Selection at age 11[1] as % of existing nursing staff resources	0%

*Figure not reliable for purpose of this exercise.
[1]Not one of our recommendations, but included for comparison purposes.

CONCLUSIONS AND POINTS FOR DISCUSSION

7.13 The decline in the school population which will occur over the next ten years will undoubtedly release resources in medical and school health nursing staff. In theory, at least, there is potential for perhaps 10% of existing medical and 12% of nursing staff resources to be devoted to new or modified school health activities. Perhaps 5% of existing medical staff resources will also be released by introducing a selective examination at school leaving, but nursing staff resources are likely to remain unaffected by this.

7.14 The cost of implementing the proposal to make special arrangements for the health surveillance of children at playgroups and day nurseries is likely to be about 15% of existing medical staff and 6% of existing nursing staff resources. The recommendation for nurse-pupil interviews might also cost about 6% of existing nursing staff resources.

7.15 We considered that a number of our recommendations are unquantifiable or have only marginal cost implications. Most of these recommendations relate to general improvements in the school health service. Taken individually the resource implications of these recommendations may be marginal, but their combined effect may well be considerable.

7.16 There is an apparent balance between the medical staffing costs of implementing the main proposals and the resources released by population change and the introduction of selective examination at school leaving age. A similar balance could be achieved for nursing staff at a marginal cost—say 2% of existing nursing staff resources. The balance between the cost of recommendations and the resources released by population change, however, would depend on the successful redeployment of staff. In our view, redeployment of staff resources released by population change would present many difficulties and would almost certainly not be fully achieved. In addition the balance takes account neither of the cost of the improvements in the school health service recommended by us nor of the cost of the increase in staffing in some health boards to meet existing demands on the service.

7.17 In considering priorities for the implementation of our recommendations during the period up to 1986 we have selected eight options. Each option assumes that selective examination will be introduced at school leaving age. If this recommendation is not proceeded with, each of the medical staff cost figures will be increased by 5% of existing resources. We have also assumed that if our recommendations to secure improvements in the school health service are proceeded with, these will absorb all the resources released by population change. The eight options are summarised in Tables 3 and 4 but these tables do not provide every possible permutation of recommendations.

Table 3—Net cost of 8 options for the implementation of health surveillance group recommendations

	Option A	Option B	Option C	Option D	Option E	Option F	Option G	Option H
Recommendation to extend examination to playgroup and day nursery children	Implement	Implement	—	—	—	—	—	—
Recommendation to introduce nurse pupil interviews	Implement	—	Implement	Implement	Implement	Implement	—	—
Recommendation to use resources released by population change for generalised improvements	Implement	Implement	Implement	—	—	—	Implement	—
Recommendation to introduce a selective examination at school leaving	*Implement*	*Implement*	*Implement*	*Implement*	*Implement*	*Implement*	*Implement*	*Implement*
Nursing cost of option as % of existing cost	12%	6%	6%	2% to 7%*	−4% to +1%*	−4% to +1%*	0%	saving* up to 10%
as estimated No. of new posts	(48)	(24)	(24)	(8 to 20)*	(−14 to +4)*	(−14 to +4)*	(0)	*saving* up to 20 posts*
Medical Staff costs of option as % of existing cost	10%	10%	0%	0% to 5%*	0% to 5%*	saving* up to 10%	0%	saving* up to 10%
as estimated No. of new posts	(20)	(20)	(0)	(0 to 10)*	(0 to 10)*	(*savings* up to 20 posts)	(0)	(*saving* up to 20 posts)

Table 4—Financial cost of 8 options for the implementation of health surveillance group recommendations

	Option A	Option B	Option C	Option D	Option E	Option F	Option G	Option H
Recommendation to extend examination to playgroup and day nursery children	Implement	Implement	—	Implement	Implement	—	—	—
Recommendation to introduce nurse pupil interviews	Implement	—	Implement	Implement	—	Implement	—	—
Recommendation to use resources released by population change for generalised improvements	Implement	Implement	Implement	—	—	—	Implement	—
Recommendation to introduce a selective examination at school leaving	*Implement*	*Implement*	*Implement*	*Implement*	*Implement*	*Implement*	*Implement*	*Implement*
Total Financial Cost Including Support Staff, Costs (pa at 1978/79 prices) £'000	495	380	114	38 to 228 *	−67 to 152 *	−333 to 19 *	NIL	−361 to NIL *

*Range results from uncertainties about redeployment of resources released by population change.

31

Chapter 8 Summary of recommendations; Priorities for change

8.1 In this chapter we summarise the recommendations which we have made in earlier chapters and, in the light of resource implications, discuss priorities for change.

SUMMARY OF RECOMMENDATIONS

Pre-school surveillance

8.2 Until a universal developmental screening programme can be implemented, special arrangements should be made to extend health surveillance to those groups of children identifiable by their attendance at nursery schools, play-groups and day nurseries. (Para. 3.4)

8.3 For all such children records should be examined to ensure that developmental screening is up to date. If it is not known to be so, with the parents' consent, the appropriate developmental screening examination should be undertaken as soon as possible. (Para. 3.5)

8.4 An annual review of all children attending nursery schools and, where possible, playgroups should be undertaken by a member of the nursing team. (Para. 3.6)

Surveillance in school

Medical examinations

8.5 All children should be medically examined during their first year at primary school. The examinations should be undertaken as soon as possible after school entry if there is no adequate record of developmental screening; otherwise it should be delayed until sufficient time has elapsed to enable the teacher to form an impression of the child's physical, emotional and intellectual development. (Paras. 3.8, 3.9)

8.6 The general practitioner should be informed of these and each subsequent examination and invited to contribute any relevant medical information. (Paras. 3.8, 3.11, 3.14)

8.7 Information about the child's present and previous health should be sought from the parents by means of a questionnaire prior to all medical examinations and reviews. Particular attention should be paid to those children whose parents do not respond. (Paras. 3.8, 3.9)

8.8 There should be a selective examination of children before entry to secondary school and in the year prior to leaving school. (Paras. 3.10, 3.14)

8.9 The selection process should include a review of the child's school medical records, including the nurse's report, and of information obtained from parents, teachers, the general practitioner and other professional staff. (Para. 3.11)

8.10 An examination should be carried out in any case in the absence of any other indication, if this is requested by the parents, or, in the case of school leavers, by the pupil. (Para. 3.14)

8.11 When programming sessions, at least 20 minutes should be allocated to each of the principal school medical examinations, exclusive of the time required for documentation. (Para. 3.28)

Height and weight
8.12 Height and weight should be measured by the school nurse, annually for primary and also for secondary pupils but on a selective basis. The results should be entered on percentile charts. (Para. 3.19)

Health care interview
8.13 A personal interview with each pupil should be held annually by the school nurse. (Para. 3.20)

Vision
8.14 All children should be screened for visual defects as soon as possible after school entry and again at the ages of 7–8, 11 and prior to school leaving. (Para. 3.22)

8.15 Colour vision should be tested at age 11. When the presence of a colour defect seems to conflict with a preference for a particular career, a detailed colour vision examination should be made. (Para. 3.23)

Hearing
8.16 Screening for hearing defects by sweep audiometry should be performed at school entry and at age 8 years. (Para. 3.24)

Cleanliness
8.17 Examinations for cleanliness and for possible infestation should be undertaken at least once a year or more frequently at the discretion of the school nurse, who should be responsible for the supervision of auxiliary staff recruited for this purpose. (Para. 3.25)

Foot defects
8.18 Children's feet should be inspected by the school nurse at the time of the annual interview, and children with foot problems further referred. (Para. 3.26)

Special examinations
8.19 A special examination should be performed whenever it is indicated by information received from a doctor, nurse, teacher, educational psychologist, social worker, parent or pupil. (Para. 3.27)

8.20 A special examination or other investigation such as a home visit by the health visitor should, unless contra-indicated, be automatically arranged after a period of school absence over four weeks. Similar action should be considered if repeated short absences from school are occurring. (Para. 3.27)

Application to special groups
8.21 Priority should be given to the extension of the surveillance programme to children in List D Schools and grant-aided schools and independent for handicapped children. (Para. 4.2)

8.22 The school health service should be extended to other grant-aided and independent schools and this should be undertaken by or under the supervision of health boards. (Para. 4.4)

Follow-up of non-attending children
8.23 Children who fail to attend routine health surveillance sessions should be followed up positively and visited at home if necessary. (Para. 4.5)

Other measures
8.24 On claiming child benefit, there should be a requirement to notify any change of address. (Para. 4.7)

Access to health advice
8.25 Parents and pupils should have ready access to the advice of both the school doctor and nurse. The means of contacting either should be made known to parents and pupils. In most circumstances the school nurse should be the first point of contact. (Paras. 5.6, 5.7)

Interchange of information
8.26 Every school should have a named school doctor, nurse and health visitor. (Para. 6.3)

8.27 The named doctor should visit the school sufficiently frequently to be known personally to the teaching staff. (Paras. 6.3, 6.5)

8.28 The named nurse should visit all schools for which she has responsibility not less frequently than once per week. (Para. 6.4)

8.29 There should be a recognised procedure for ensuring that the findings of health personnel involved in screening examinations are brought to the attention of the appropriate health and educational staff. (Para. 6.8)

8.30 The school doctor should be informed of the referral of children to the educational psychologist, child psychiatrist or child guidance service. (Para. 6.10)

8.31 The Community Medicine Specialist with responsibility for child health should be the person in each health board responsible for requesting and receiving school health records from outwith the area. (Para. 6.11)

Research recommendations

8.32 A national research exercise should be mounted to validate the use of selection by the examination of a control group of children at both the ages at which selective examination is recommended. (Paras. 3.13, 3.16)

8.33 Studies should be undertaken to compare the relative cost effectiveness of the visual screening of pre-school children carried out by orthoptists with screening carried out by doctors and health visitors during the course of their routine contacts with children. (Para. 3.21)

8.34 A study should be mounted to assess the cost effectiveness of staff intensive programmes for the follow up of defaulters. (Para. 4.6)

PRIORITIES FOR CHANGE

8.35 In the light of the estimates of the staff implications of the implementation of our recommendations, we considered the net cost of implementing various combinations of recommendations. These combinations are presented as eight options in Table 3 in Chapter 7. Clearly the Table does not provide every possible permutation of recommendations since we consider that a selective examination should be introduced at school leaving irrespective of which of the other recommendations are to be adopted. At the same time, we made the assumption that, where a decision is taken to secure general improvements in the school health service, this would be met most efficiently by taking up resources released by the projected decline in the school population up to 1986.

8.36 We have no doubt that, in the light of the results of the quantification study, we must recommend that our three principal recommendations detailed in paragraph 7.3 should be accepted, and that any resources released by the projected decline in the school population should be used to secure general improvements in the school health service along the lines of our other recommendations. (Option A in Table 3.)

Financial cost of recommendations

8.37 The model which we developed takes no account of the consequences for numbers of administrative staff or of changing the medical and nursing staff complement. Each of the eight options for the implementation of our recommendation summarised in Table 3 has been costed at 1978/79 prices by Scottish Office Accountancy Services with an allowance for supporting staff costs and a note on this costing appears at Appendix E. The estimates of the total cost at 1978/79 prices of each of the eight options is shown in Table 4 in Chapter 7.

Conclusions

8.38 Although there are likely to be savings of resources resulting from the projected decrease in the school population, in some areas part at least of these savings will require to be directed towards bringing the school health service up to existing requirements. In addition, there are many recommendations which individually have no major resource implications but which taken collectively will have a significant cost. If these recommendations are lost to the school health service because of lack of resources much of the value of our report will disappear. Further, as we have already indicated, the optimum benefits of our recommendations depend on the existence of an effective pre-school screening service and we realise that this too may well involve additional resources. We envisage, therefore, that any savings of resources which may arise from changes in school population in the future will be fully absorbed in achieving a properly integrated school health service, with all the pre-school screening and the school age health surveillance which such a service entails. In these circumstances additional resources will be required to secure an increased nursing presence in schools and annual nurse pupil interviews. Increased resources will also be required so that special arrangements can be made to carry out health surveillance in playgroups, although whether these resources need to be made available to the school health service would depend on organisational arrangements.

Part II
Children with handicap

Chapter 9   Introduction

9.1 The objective of the Health Service for school children is to apply the professional resources available to it in such a way that 'no child is prevented by ill health from obtaining an education appropriate to his age, ability and aptitude and that all children leave school in the best possible state of physical and emotional health' (chapter 16, paragraph 6 of the Brotherston Report[6]). This part of our report on the school health service relates that objective to handicapped children.

9.2 For the purpose of this report it is important to be clear as to what we mean by the two terms 'handicap' and 'disability'. Chapter 14 of the Court Report[7] recognises the need for identification and management of developmental disorders, medical and surgical conditions in children. Paragraph 14.2 of that report defines the two terms 'handicap' and 'disability' in a manner with which we do not entirely agree. In our view, 'disability' in a child refers to a mental or physical disorder which interferes with function. The word 'handicap' implies that the disability from which the child suffers adversely affects his activities, opportunities and expectations. Thus a serious disability could, in a given case, produce only a minor handicap to the child's educational performances. The reverse could be equally true.

9.3 In this report when we speak of 'assessment of a handicapped child' we mean the procedures for examining identified disabilities, for evaluating any resultant handicap(s) not only in relation to health but also education, and for making appropriate plans for treatment or care. Assessment is a continuing process whether it is carried out as a formal inter-professional matter, or through routine but informal contacts between professional workers. Assessment and the continuing management of the handicapped child are one composite procedure which should be the same regardless of the particular agency, whether health or education, responsible for the child at the time. The main stages of assessment are:

Identification of the problem;

Collation of relevant information including any previous findings which may be available;

Investigation and clinical examination;

Consideration and evaluation of the child's whole history jointly by professional workers in the relevant disciplines;

Decision on treatment and management for the child;

Re-assessment where appropriate.

9.4 Co-operation across a broad professional front will be essential if the needs of the handicapped child are to be correctly identified and fully met on a continuing basis. In order to be successful, assessment procedures, particularly in relation to the continuing management of the child's special problems and needs, must be both flexible and acceptable to the full range of professional workers involved. The success of assessment depends on the collaboration of general practitioners, school doctors, community nursing staff, medical specialists, and members of other professions, notably teachers, psychologists, social workers and remedial therapists.

9.5 Although in this report we concentrate on handicap in the context of a child's education, we do not confine ourselves to the assessment of children of school age. The importance of the early detection of disability was emphasised in Chapter 3 of Part I of this report, which deals with health surveillance. The corollary of early detection must be early action to assess and meet the needs which are revealed.

References

[6]*Towards an Integrated Child Health Service.* A report of a joint Working Party on the integration of medical work. Chairman: Sir John Brotherston, Scottish Home and Health Department, Edinburgh, HMSO, 1973.

[7]*Fit for the Future.* The report of the Committee on Child Health Services. Chairman: Professor S. D. M. Court, London, HMSO, 1976, Cmnd. 6684.

Chapter 10   Prevalence of disability

10.1 Because of the paucity of routine national data relating to the prevalence of disability in children, estimates must be based on data from special studies. There are considerable differences between existing studies both in the groups of children surveyed and in the definitions of disability adopted. In consequence, the results of these studies cannot always be regarded as strictly comparable. For this reason any estimates of prevalence based on the aggregation of data from a variety of sources must be viewed with considerable caution. The shortage of available data points to the need for research on the prevalence of disability.

10.2 Estimates of prevalence of disability do not by themselves provide a basis for estimating the proportion of the child population requiring assessment because, firstly, more than one disability may be present in the same child, and secondly, there will be many children who require assessment but in whom no disability will ultimately be found. Amongst this latter group there will be many children who suffer from social disadvantages.

10.3 Despite these limitations, estimates of the prevalence of disabilities in children based on current evidence are of value in providing guidelines on the proportion of the child population actually or potentially handicapped because of a disability. We have thought it helpful to give some consideration to the data available so as to give an indication of the extent of the problems.

10.4 The Court Committee estimated that of children aged 0–15 the proportion who would need special health care because of physical, motor, visual, hearing and communication or learning disorders would be about 9% of a given child population. These estimates were based on an assessment of data from a variety of sources including a study of handicap of children in Livingston (Bain, 1973)[8], a study of severe speech defects in a national sample of 7-year-olds (Sheridan and Peckham, 1973)[9], studies of mental handicap in children (eg Birch, 1970)[10] as well as the results of the comprehensive survey of 9–11 year-olds carried out in the Isle of Wight (Rutter *et al.*, 1970)[11] and a study of school entrants in Newcastle upon Tyne (Miller *et al.*, 1974)[12].

10.5 The Court Committee's estimates relate specifically to children needing special health care, but their Report stresses that they exclude children handicapped by psychiatric disorder. The Committee stated that at a conservative estimate between 5 and 10% of all children will be affected by some form of psychiatric disorder in a single year. Many of these children are also likely to display evidence of developmental, social, or educational handicap.

10.6 Although the Court estimates relate ostensibly to England and Wales, the sources quoted include both Scottish data (Bain, 1973) and national data (Sheridan and Peckham, 1973) and in the absence of evidence to the contrary it seems reasonable to assume that the estimates would be just as applicable in Scotland as they are in England and Wales.

10.7 The Court Committee do not state the assumptions which they have made in reaching their conclusions as to the prevalence of disability, and we have not found it possible to reconstruct their estimates from the sources given. Our own examination of the same sources suggests that a range of estimates could be made depending on which of the data contained in these sources are included in the analysis and how these are used. For this reason it is our view that the Court estimates provide only a general guide to the prevalence of disabling conditions. At Appendix F there is set out an estimate of prevalence of handicapping conditions, derived from various sources.

10.8 If disability is taken to include educational backwardness, then it may be estimated on the basis of the Isle of Wight study that perhaps 16% of children will have some form of disability. This estimate corresponds well with the estimate made by the Warnock Committee[13], on the basis of the results of the National Child Development Study, that 17% of children would require some form of special educational provision during any one year.

10.9 While educational placement is an important aspect of assessment, the main burden of assessment work will relate to the general aspects of the care and management of handicapped children. This is underlined by the fact that, on the basis of recent statistics for Scotland, only a small minority of children (13,680 in 1976/77) with disability, as defined by the Court or the Warnock Committees, required education in special schools or classes.

10.10 Our examination of data relating to the prevalence of disability was initially undertaken as a step towards estimating the volume of assessment work which will be required in carrying out our recommendations. We have come to recognise that, apart from the lack of definitive data, the translation of information on disability into any calculation of assessment workload will present major problems. We return to this matter in Chapter 17.

References

[8]Bain, D. J. G. *Health Centre Practice in Livingston New Town.* Health Bulletin, 31(6) November, 1973.

[9]Sheridan, M. D. and Peckham, C. S. *Hearing and Speech at Seven.* Special Education, 62(2), 1973.

[10]Birch, H. G. et al. *Mental Subnormality in the Community.* Baltimore, Williams and Wilkins, 1970.

[11]Rutter, M., Tizard, J., and Whitmore, K. *Education, Health and Behaviour.* London, Longman, 1970.

[12]Miller, F. J. W. et al. *School Years in Newcastle upon Tyne 1952-1962.* London, Oxford University Press, 1974.

[13]*Special Educational Needs.* Report of the Committee of Enquiry into the Education of Handicapped Children and Young People. Chairman: Mrs H. M. Warnock, London, HMSO, 1978. Cmnd. 7212.

Chapter 11 The wider context of assessment

11.1 As a preliminary to the detailed consideration of assessment, we now consider the wider background against which the need for assessment arises. This includes the responsibilities of the different statutory agencies involved, and, the way in which these may affect the conduct of inter-professional assessment.

11.2 In health terms, assessment is a linking process, starting with health surveillance and the other services which may detect handicap, and proceeding to arrangements for treatment or care. It may extend beyond the normal process of inter-professional consultation, because the object of assessment is to consider the total situation of the child and to call upon whatever range of profes sional resources may be necessary to evaluate his needs and how best to meet them. The degree of consultation involved will vary widely from case to case. A multi-disciplinary approach will be employed only as and when circumstances require. (We return to this matter in paragraph 11.15.) This approach frequently involves collaboration between the health service and the education and social work services.

Interrelation of health, education and social work services

11.3 The existence of health, education and social work services, each concerned with different aspects of the welfare of the child, poses problems for the organisation of inter-professional assessment. For example, there should be arrangements which provide a basis for decision-taking specifically related to the statutory duties of each agency. Each professional may well have an important but quite separate contribution to make towards assessment, not related to the statutory responsibility of the agency which that professional serves. The question of clinical or other professional responsibility for the child may be a complicating factor.

11.4 Though health boards and social work and education authorities have quite separate statutory responsibilities in relation to children and operate services through staff who are, for the most part, members of separate professional groups, these agencies have substantial common interests with regard to the physical, emotional and social development of children. Children who have health problems will frequently require special management in school. On the other hand, children with educational or health problems will not necessarily require social work attention on an individual basis. Nevertheless there is a general responsibility[14] on regional authorities to provide a social welfare service to assist persons in need. In addition, they have specific responsibilities in certain circumstances for individual children, deriving from their powers and duties [15] to provide voluntary or compulsory measures of care for children on a residential or non-residential basis. Situations calling for these measures may arise quite independently of child health problems. At the same time, the need for care can, and frequently does, have a health component, as in the case of the very young and others who are subject to, or at risk of, neglect or physical abuse.

11.5 The procedure for 'educational ascertainment' laid down in the Education (Scotland) Acts 1962 and 1969 requires an education authority to identify those children of school age living in their area who may be in need of special education; to arrange for such children to undergo medical and psychological examination; to take a formal decision regarding the child's educational needs; and to communicate this to the child's parents. In reaching its decision the authority is required to take into account any other reports or information which it is able to obtain with regard to the ability or aptitude of the child. This will frequently involve multi-disciplinary assessment, with the education authority being guided by any recommendation resulting therefrom. The statute also recognises the need for early identification of handicap by providing a separate discretionary power to take similar action in the cases of children who are over the age of two but under school age. There is an increasing trend in some areas for the education authority to exercise its ascertainment duties informally in consultation with the parents and without involving the full statutory procedures.

11.6 We are aware that detailed guidance has been issued by the Scottish Education Department in the past on the ascertainment of maladjusted children and those with impaired hearing or vision, based studies by expert groups in the various fields concerned. This advice has emphasised the need for multi-disciplinary assessment following on the identification of a specific handicap, and multi-professional teams have been set up in some areas under education authority arrangements for this purpose. The recommendations which we make in Chapters 12 and 13 assume that it will be possible to avoid the duplication involved in having separate multi-disciplinary assessment teams set up by health boards and education authorities. The implications of this in terms of consultation between health boards and local authorities are considered in Chapter 16.

11.7 The common interest of health and education services in the healthy development of children begins before the entry of the child into the formal educational system. As already mentioned, the education authority has powers to ascertain the future needs of pre-school children for special education, and also to provide nursery education for children of pre-school years. Educational ascertainment of children below school age does not need to be a formal process. The education authority may adopt a variety of roles in planning the education of the child and, in collaboration with the parents, in providing some early educational experience in the child's home. The full benefit of pre-school health surveillance depends not only on the health input, but also on the interest of the education authority in the results obtained and on its willingness to commit skilled professional resources to help the child even before he enters the educational system formally.

11.8 There is a growing awareness, as highlighted in the Warnock Report (*see* para. 5.25), that assessment is a continuing process in which, especially in the case of younger children, care, management and education are essential components. We agree with this view and recommend that, wherever possible, health and education authorities should combine to provide centres in which care, management, education and parent counselling are provided as an integral part of assessment.

11.9 While the health and educational services are concerned with all handicapped children individually, the nature of the demand on social work services will vary from case to case as already indicated. A poor quality of family and neighbourly support may suggest a need for social work assessment and help. We recommend that health professionals should collaborate with social workers in assessing the situation of families with handicapped children, taking into account the needs and demands of the family as well as those of the child. The relationship between the two professional groups will depend upon the degree and timing of the involvement of each. There will be many cases in which social needs will predominate, and in these the social worker should play the leading role. Such cases will include emotional crises where strong feelings impair the family's caring capability, or social crises where urgent arrangements need to be made for the physical care of the child. Case conferences should be organised where appropriate so as to achieve the collaboration desirable amongst all the professionals who are involved with the family.

11.10 It is relevant to distinguish between, on the one hand, developmental or other health assessment of the handicapped child where the factors involved are primarily physical or psychological, and, on the other hand, assessment of the child whose difficulty relates more to his external social situation. At the extremes, it is possible to distinguish between 'the handicapped child' with whom the health and education services will be primarily involved, and 'the child in need of care' for whom the social work services will assume statutory and largely separate responsibility. Recognition of this distinction is implicit in the advice given by the Social Work Services Group of the Scottish Education Department to local authorities in 1971, based on the report of a working party[16] which studied the arrangements for the assessment of children by social work departments in the light of the introduction at that time of the system of Children's Hearings. Inter-professional assessment teams under the control of social work departments have been established in some parts of Scotland in response to this advice.

11.11 The proposals which we suggest for a multi-disciplinary assessment system shared between health and education services will not in our view cut across the arrangements of the social work service for carrying out assessments for their own purposes. Very close collaboration between the two systems will be essential, and, with that end in view, we make proposals in Chapters 13 and 14 for reciprocal membership of the two assessment teams. It must be accepted, however, that there will be a substantial overlap between the two assessment systems. Handicapped children may be in trouble because of difficult behaviour; they may suffer parental neglect or even abuse; non-accidental injury may result in physical or intellectual handicap. Many children have complex problems in physical, psychological and social terms, and these may be among the most difficult of all children to help. Good understanding between the members of the different services as to their over-lapping responsibilities and concerns is essential in order to avoid the wasteful use of professional skills and to minimise confusion within the families involved. We recommend that the two systems should be monitored in order to evaluate the contribution of each to the assessment of children with complex but related difficulties. In our view this monitoring should be primarily a health service responsibility.

11.12 It might be possible for a comprehensive assessment system, designed primarily to meet the needs of the health and education services, to be extended to cover the requirements of social work services—all three services employing one single multi-disciplinary team. We consider that such a system will probably be practicable only in some rural areas with small populations. Appropriate health boards should be encouraged to test this proposal.

The multi-disciplinary approach

11.13 Throughout this part of our report, we emphasise the importance of a multi-disciplinary approach to the assessment of handicap in children, and subsequent management. The development of an integrated approach by a number of workers of different but related disciplines has proved particularly advantageous with regard to the emotional disorders and handicapping conditions of childhood. Traditionally, the child psychiatrist has worked closely with the psychologist and social worker; he has also co-operated with the teacher, nurse, occupational and speech therapists. More recently the paediatrician, especially when concerned with developmental assessment and the management of handicaps, both physical and mental, has worked closely with all of these disciplines.

11.14 There are good reasons for this close collaboration. A comprehensive assessment (a broader term than 'diagnosis') of handicap calls for an appraisal, both at the time and subsequently, of how this affects the child's general health, capacity for learning, social development and ability to cope with the demands of ordinary living. In any assessment it is also important to have regard to the stresses which the parents and those who care for and seek to educate the child must necessarily experience. No one discipline can aspire to complete knowledge of, and competence in, all these aspects of the child's life.

11.15 In relatively straightforward situations of single handicap, where the child and the parents are co-operative and well-motivated, the clinical task may be undertaken by one specialist with appropriate assistance from other specialist colleagues; eg in the case of hearing loss the paediatrician will be assisted both by the audiometrician's report on hearing, and also by the psychologist's assessment of developmental status. Where more complex or multiple handicaps exist, and especially where there are also difficult social or family relationships, a multi-disciplinary team approach is likely to be necessary. This means that the tasks of assessment and management are shared by a closely knit group of experts, who, by establishing an intimate professional relationship over a period of time, have acquired a collective skill in working with children and their families.

11.16 The sharing of information and the co-ordination of effort are the most elementary steps in team-work. As an extension of this aspect of teamwork it may be advantageous for two or more members of a group of professional workers to take part in a joint examination of the child. A multi-disciplinary team aims to develop a common pool of expertise, a capacity for reaching decisions by consensus, and a flexible outlook in counselling. This kind of approach will inevitably cross traditional professional boundaries and it will have implications for decision-taking where different professional responsibilities are involved.

References

[14]Social Work (Scotland) Act 1968 Section 12 and Chronically Sick and Disabled Persons (Scotland) Act 1972 Section 1.
[15]Social Work (Scotland) Act 1968 Section 15 and Part III.
[16]*Assessment of Children.* Social Work Services Group, Scottish Education Department, Edinburgh, 1971.

Chapter 12 The handicapped child at home and at school

12.1 Assessment involves a decision about how best a child suffering from handicap can be supported and his difficulties managed. The objective is to enable the child to live and be educated in, or as closely as possible to, his own family and the community of which his family forms a part. We therefore turn in this Chapter to consider the needs of the handicapped child in terms of physical and other provision to enable him to cope, both at home and at school, with the wide range of problems which may arise as a result of his handicap. We also consider the role of the parents and teachers, as they have the immediate care of the child for most of his early life. Concern with the continuing health surveillance of handicapped children leads us to consider the usefulness of handicap registers.

Facilities in schools

12.2 It is generally agreed that a handicapped child should attend the local primary and secondary schools so far as this is practicable and in his best interests. How far this can be achieved depends upon a number of factors such as the degree of disability, the child's attitude to his handicap, his temperament, his ability and educational attainments, the attitude of his parents and the resources of the school. It may be easier to apply this policy in the case of some disabilities than others. In cases of severe mental handicap, profound deafness or blindness, for instance, the limitations on what can be achieved are obvious. Some children with severe and/or multiple disabilities will always require the special teaching and other facilities which are only available in special schools, whether day or residential.

12.3 The type of accommodation available in any particular primary and secondary school is often a vital factor when deciding whether the handicapped child can or cannot be admitted. Section 8 of the Chronically Sick and Disabled Persons Act 1970 requires that provision for the needs of disabled persons be made in new educational establishments insofar as it is both practical and reasonable in the circumstances. The Scottish Education Department has since recommended[17] that in the design of new schools consideration should be given to the provision of facilities which would enable a greater number of physically handicapped children to attend an ordinary local school rather than a special school, and has indicated the kinds of measure which might be adopted, such as the provision of ramps, hand rails and special toilet facilities. The circular pointed out that although Section 8 applied only to new educational establishments it was hoped that authorities would also keep in view the practicability of adapting some existing buildings to meet the needs of the disabled.

12.4 We comment in Chapter 15 on the need for adequate accommodation in schools to enable health professionals (including a wide range of para-medical and other specialists) to carry out their functions. We mention there the needs of the school assessment team for accommodation. The presence of increasing numbers of handicapped children in a school has implications for the accommodation and facilities which will be required for visiting specialists. We recommend that education authorities should take steps to ensure that both in special schools, and in those catering for a significant number of handicapped children, there should be adequate accommodation for specialist visiting services, over and above the normal requirements of the school doctor and nurse and the school dental service. In this connection we draw attention to the advice given by the Scottish Education Department in 1975[18] on the different types of accommodation required by visiting specialist services.

12.5 We recommend that the minimum accommodation for school health staff in all but the smallest schools should be a consultation room for exclusive use by the school doctor and nurse, with space there or elsewhere for storage of school health records (which are confidential) unless arrangements have been made for records to be kept in health board premises. The need to secure records against the activities of vandals is important. Beyond this, we accept that the provision of separate accommodation (eg for medical examination and dental treatment), while being highly desirable, may have to depend on the size of the school. Accommodation shared with 'non-health' staff is bound to give rise to recurrent difficulties. The continuing decline in school populations should release some of the space required to improve the accommodation position in existing as well as new schools. We agree that the responsibility for providing basic facilities should continue to rest with education authorities acting under guidance from the Secretary of State as regards the design and standards of school buildings. This will not, however, bring about the much needed improvement in standards in existing schools which cater for numbers of handicapped children. We recommend that health boards should be enabled more readily to secure exclusive use of accommodation of the standard which health staff require in both new and existing schools. One means to this end would be for health boards to rent accommodation in existing schools and adapt it for their purposes. Alternatively health boards might pay the capital cost of any accommodation in new schools which is supplementary to that prescribed in design guidance. This is a suitable subject for discussion by the joint liaison committees referred to in Chapter 16.

Roles of parents and teachers

12.6 Professionals who are involved with the handicapped child must always bear in mind that it is his parents who have the principal caring responsibility for him. Even when the parents are not able to cope unaided, they should be involved as soon as the handicap is identified both in planning for the care of the child, and in his subsequent assessment. At the time of the initial diagnosis, they need to be helped to come to terms with the situation which is revealed by assessment. This support is likely to be a continuing necessity which will involve particularly the general practitioner, the psychiatrist and the social worker. They must be kept informed of all aspects of the child's management and encouraged to share in decisions and care (though clearly the extent of this will depend both on the parents and on the type of the handicap). The effects of the handicap on the parents and siblings must be watched closely because of the stress which they may suffer. The primary care team will be involved in this task. In some cases the therapist may be involved, but in most cases the immediate supervision of the family is likely to fall upon the health visitor or social worker, depending on the particular arrangements for home visiting and family support.

12.7 A close working relationship between parents and professionals is essential if each is to be able to play his proper part in helping the child. Parents should be involved in and kept informed about assessment or other discussions which take place regarding the care or treatment of the handicapped child. It is essential that the professionals involved in such situations should decide which of them is to keep the parents informed and which is to provide any counselling and support which the parents may require. (In Chapter 14 we deal with the position of parents in relation to multi-disciplinary assessments carried out by the district assessment team.)

12.8 Teachers share with parents the main burden of responsibility in caring for the needs of handicapped children of school age. The health problems of such children, for example a child with convulsions, may become an emergency which calls for prompt action. We recommend that all teachers should have training in such matters as part of pre-service and in-service courses. This will extend to the use and custody of the drugs which are used in treating handicapped children. If possible these courses should be given by a doctor or nurse or health visitor actively involved in educational medicine. School doctors should be responsible for arranging in-service training for teachers and other relevant staff to update their knowledge of health matters.

12.9 In the field of health education, handicapped children have particular health needs which may call for a special approach and a change of emphasis. Sex education and preparation for parenthood are seen as important but neglected topics which merit special consideration in health education programmes designed for handicapped children. In addition to such general health education, the handicapped child may require counselling on an individual basis.

12.10 Teachers need up-to-date information on local resources which are relevant to the care and management of children with handicap. They require to know where, and to whom, they can turn for assistance should the need arise; this is especially true in large areas where there is a multiplicity of services. Leaflets containing such data should be drawn up by health boards and distributed to all teachers. The Scottish Health Education Unit has recently produced a guide[19] containing comprehensive, but simply presented, first aid measures and health information about conditions with which the teacher may be confronted. This is an interesting document which will assist discussion of this matter. We recommend that health education units of health boards should assume responsibility for the provision of any such documents for which a need may be identified locally.

12.11 The school doctor has an important part to play in keeping both the head teacher and classroom teacher informed about the special needs of individual handicapped children; this is particularly important when the child starts school. The health section of the pupil's Progress Record Card is of great importance and it should be the joint responsibility of the school doctor and the head teacher to see that it is completed and kept up to date. The Record Card when kept up to date will be a useful addition to verbal communication. In primary and special schools teachers readily take on 'caring' responsibilities for health matters, including the administration of some drugs. This practice should be encouraged, provided that adequate nursing and medical support is available. In secondary schools the aim should be to encourage handicapped children, like the other children, to become responsible for their own health and hygiene, although they will still need continuing support from the school nurse or the guidance teacher.

12.12 Occasions will arise when teachers will require day-to-day assistance in coping with the special needs of handicapped children. The level of assistance will depend upon the number of such children involved in a given situation and the type of management problems which they present. We think that in many instances auxiliaries with appropriate in-service training could be of great help, provided that the back-up of a qualified visiting nursing service is available. We recommend that the question of such appointments should be discussed jointly between health and education authorities as to local needs and the exact nature of the duties to be performed.

Special requirements: aids and equipment, recreation provision etc

12.13 We now refer to various types of special provision which will normally be found where handicapped children are being educated or otherwise cared for in a well-provided environment, but which for one reason or another may be neglected when the child is placed in the community alongside children with lesser disability or no disability at all. Therapists have an important role to play in the provision of aids and equipment and of recreation in all circumstances.

12.14 Health boards and local authorities arc both involved in ensuring the provision of such aids, the ready availability and the appropriateness of which are of prime importance for any disabled person. Confusion, however, has sometimes arisen in the minds of professional staff and the public about the division of responsibility between them. This matter was highlighted in both the Mair Report on Medical Rehabilitation[20] and Baroness Sharp's Report on the Mobility of Physically Disabled People[21]. We endorse the advice given in a circular issued by the Scottish Home and Health Department in October 1976[22] inviting health boards and local authorities to work out local procedures for the supply of all necessary aids and equipment. We recommend that, where local procedures have not already been agreed and put into operation, action on this important matter should be taken without delay.

12.15 Play, recreation and holidays are essential to stimulate and encourage the mental, physical and emotional development of mentally and physically handicapped children. In the case of handicapped children in residential schools, whether the child has a home to return to or not, suitable weekend and holiday arrangements should be provided. Holiday camps afford a valuable opportunity to assess the capabilities of the children away from the school environment, and they foster the child's own feelings of independence. We recommend that the provision of medical and nurse staff in such situations should be a school health service commitment. The type of staff and the numbers involved will depend on the needs of the children concerned.

12.16 Some handicapped children are not in the care either of their parents or of foster parents, and the social work department may have parental responsibility for them. Some of these children may be in children's homes and some may be, temporarily or otherwise, in hospital placements. In addition to educational, medical and nursing attention, such children will need the equivalent of a home base where there will be a continuity of 'caring' by somebody experienced in meeting the social and emotional needs of children who do not have the benefit of a family upbringing. 'Caring' in this context should include planning for holidays and other excursions which will serve to enlarge the child's horizons. Assessment teams considering the situation of such children will require to have the benefit of the views of whoever is acting *in loco parentis* for the time being.

12.17 Recreational needs will vary widely according to the age and circumstances of the child. Parents and others involved in meeting these needs may require expert guidance and also assistant with equipment. Toy libraries providing a service for handicapped children are valuable in helping parents to develop the potential of their child through play. It is important for members of the primary care team to recognise the value of suitable play, to know where expert advice is available and to enlist appropriate voluntary help.

12.18 There is a great need for short-stay accommodation for handicapped children, to enable parents to have a much needed holiday. Provision is especially necessary in cases of family crisis; such needs will arise at short notice. Trained childminders may be of great help to the parents of handicapped children of school age, not only for the benefit of the children but also to give their families a respite from the burden of caring for them. In this field we recommend that education authorities should be asked to consider the need for, and feasibility of, introducing more continuous attendance throughout the year at special schools for mentally and physically handicapped children, and that they should be asked to undertake responsibility for working out holiday activity programmes for handicapped children, using school premises as appropriate. Such programmes might necessitate staggered staff holidays and/or the employment of an entirely different group of workers, and would require careful planning. We recommend that health boards should provide health cover for the children concerned.

12.19 The provision of adequate transport facilities is essential for a large number of handicapped children, not just to get them to and from school and to clinics and hospitals but, equally important, to allow them to join with their peers in activities organised by the school outwith school premises. Problems may occur where specialist transport is required for a small number of children and additional expense will arise where escorts or attendants are required. We recommend that the provision of transport should be discussed by health boards and local authorities as part of the arrangements for liaison mentioned in Chapter 16. The use of a car should make a radical difference to the lives of the whole family of a severely handicapped child by reducing both the physical burden and the social isolation which they experience. The Family Fund, administered by the Rowntree Memorial Trust, has provided valuable help in this field. We hope that, where resources permit, social work departments in conjunction with voluntary bodies will look sympathetically at continuing and extending this form of assistance in suitable cases.

Keeping handicapped children in view

12.20 It is very important that handicapped children should have all the benefits of health surveillance in the same way as other children. In Part I of this report we have expressly stated (in Chapter 4) that the health surveillance measures which we propose are equally applicable to all children whether handicapped or not and whether in special schools or in ordinary primary or secondary schools.

12.21 We deal in Chapter 14 with the role of assessment teams in reviewing the cases of children who have already been assessed. We distinguish, in relation to the district assessment team in particular, between the cases which may call for re-assessment or review by the team itself and cases where the task may be delegated to school assessment teams. We endorse what is said in the Brotherston Report (Chapter 15, para. 12) as to the special importance of good health records where handicapped children are concerned. We draw attention to the views which we have expressed in Part IV of this report regarding the establishment and maintenance of a proper records system. We recommend that health boards, acting through the appropriate Community Medicine Specialist, should assume responsibility for maintaining, up-dating and reviewing a register at district level of children with handicap. We discuss in Chapter 14 the part which the district assessment team should play in these arrangements. The arrangements made by the education authority for recording the progress of children receiving special education will, to some extent, meet the authority's own needs where the children concerned are placed in a school under its direct control. We are in no doubt, however, that health boards must make separate arrangements for recording particulars of children with handicap and for showing their progress at regular intervals.

12.22 We are aware that the objectives of handicap registers currently maintained are concerned largely with identifying the number of children with handicapping conditions and its implications for the provision of services. We consider that the scope of handicap registers ought to be widened to provide a basis for the continuing surveillance of handicapped children. To achieve this, a handicap register should fulfil two types of function. The first type of function would operate at local level and would be:

    (a) to provide in each district a master list of children with handicap requiring special health oversight (including children for whom special educational treatment has been arranged);

    (b) to act as a check list for periodic reviews (whether by the district assessment team or otherwise);

    (c) to facilitate the transfer of information on a child moving from one area to another (eg providing appropriate notification to another health board or health district to which the child was moved);

The second type of function would operate both at local and at national level and would be:

    (d) to provide information on the prevalence of handicapping conditions which will assist in planning future provision of health, education and social work services, in monitoring trends and in epidemiological research.

12.23 We recognise that registers with these functions will achieve their maximum usefulness only if they are compiled and maintained on a common basis throughout Scotland. Questions as to how this might be achieved are complex and are not within the remit of the group. We consider, however, that a review of the scope and function of handicap registers is urgently required. Ideally such a review should extend to the interests of education and social work services. We recommend that the Scottish Home and Health Department should initiate such a review.

References

[17]Scottish Education Department, Circular No. 782, 5 February 1971. The Chronically Sick and Disabled Persons Act 1970.

[18]*Visiting Services Suites*. Scottish Education Department, Educational Building Note No. 13. Edinburgh, HMSO, 1975.

[19]*Index of First Aid and Problems for Schools*. Scottish Health Education Unit, Edinburgh, 1978.

[20]*Medical Rehabilitation: The pattern for the future*. Report of a sub-committee of the Standing Medical Advisory Committee, Scottish Health Services Council, Scottish Home and Health Department, Edinburgh, HMSO, 1972.

[21]*Mobility of Physically Disabled People*. Lady Sharp, DBE, London, HMSO, 1974.

[22]Scottish Home and Health Department, NHS Circular 1976 (GEN) 90. Provision by Health Boards and Local Authorities of Aids and Equipment for the Disabled living at home and adaptations to their homes. Edinburgh, HMSO, 1973.

Chapter 13 Framework for assessment

13.1 In this chapter we consider how a system of assessment can be established which:

a. meets the differing requirements of the health and education services as discussed in Chapter 11;

b. has ready access to the expertise of different professions and disciplines as appropriate; and

c. encourages a flexible and economical working arrangement which facilitates inter-professional communication.

13.2 Despite the need for flexibility, any assessment system will only be effective in practice if the basic principles of assessment are clear and are generally accepted by those concerned. In practice, arrangements must be tailored to fit the characteristics of individual areas and the availability of resources therein, and therefore the details of the system must be worked out locally by those involved.

Tiers of assessment

13.3 The general framework for assessment which we propose builds on existing guidance in this field and on current practice. Our proposals suggest assessment at three different 'levels', and they preserve the existing process of medical referral from the primary care network to hospital and other specialist services. The three levels are designed to meet the needs of both health and education interests. The flow diagram at Appendix G indicates the three levels of assessment (local, district and regional), the ways in which children who have been identified as having problems may 'enter the system' at either of the first two of these levels and the main patterns of referral. We envisage that assessment arrangements at local and district level should be similar throughout Scotland, whereas 'regional' assessment will involve the sophisticated diagnostic and other facilities which are available in the main paediatric and other specialist centres.

13.4 The original referrals for assessment are shown in the flow diagram as coming from individual professional workers concerned with children at the local level, including doctors in the primary care team or at school, and teachers and others who come into direct contact with children in schools. It may well be that parents will make the first move by seeking advice. The majority of referrals are likely to arise from the three usual situations in which handicap is initially detected;

    a. medical examinations (for example children of any age examined because of illness or injury).

    b. pre-school developmental screening;

    c. health surveillance within schools.

In the case of pre-school children, 'local' assessment arrangements would depend on the existence of child health clinics and health centres where a similar service is provided. In the absence of such clinics, infants and pre-school children would be referred direct to the district assessment team.

13.5 Where children are attending school or nursery school, 'local' assessment, will normally be by health and other professional workers in the school health service. This, like assessment at district level, entails some selection because there will be many children suffering from relatively straightforward conditions who can be cared for either by the primary care team or by a single professional working in consultation with colleagues in his own or another discipline. We recommend, accordingly, that school health personnel, in collaboration with colleagues in other disciplines as appropriate, should act as a school assessment team when they meet to consider the cases of children with possible handicap. We recommend that where children are attending playgroups or day nurseries at which the school health service provides health surveillance, the same arrangements should apply.

13.6 We recommend that the regular or 'core' members of the school assessment team should be the school doctor, the school nurse, a teacher with detailed knowledge of the child and the educational psychologist and social worker who have particular responsibility for the school. The general practitioner and any other member of the primary care team who knows about the child should be automatically co-opted to the team. The general practitioner should always be invited to participate in discussions on children who are his patients, as should any health visitor who is known to be in contact with the family. Similarly, assistance should be sought from any para-medical staff who may be able to contribute. We recommend that school assessment teams should meet on a regular basis because, in order to obtain the full benefits of inter-disciplinary cooperation, it is essential that there should be frequent, and not always formal meetings of the team members. The decisions of the team may well cover a wide field including special health care, or supervision at home or in the school, as well as proposals for consideration by the education department about the educational management of the child. With parental agreement the school assessment team may refer to the district assessment team any child whose problems require additional expertise for their assessment. Whilst we hope that the general practitioner who is looking after a child will attend all assessment sessions relating to the child, it is essential that all assessment decisions relating to the child should be communicated to him.

13.7 We recommend that special schools should have school assessment teams in the same way as other schools, but in their case the 'core' membership of the team should be extended to include professionals with expertise in the particular handicap concerned. These teams will have a major function to perform in the process of reassessment and review. We deal with the relationship of the school assessment team in special schools to the district assessment team in Chapter 14. We also recommend that such local teams which have a special expertise should, in addition to their work in special schools, be available to visit children with the relevant handicap who are attending local primary or secondary schools.

13.8 The arrangements for assessment above local level must necessarily be more structured. Some mention of the district assessment team must be made at this juncture in order to explain the whole framework shown in the flow diagram. (A detailed description is reserved for Chapter 14.) The district assessment team will comprise a 'core' of members working together for the major part of their time either on particular assessments or on general matters relating thereto. The 'core' members will have authority to call on the services of specialists in any of the health, education, social work or other fields as circumstances may dictate with a view to assembling the complete range of expertise requisite to the assessment being undertaken.

13.9 The assessment of some children having a rare or complex disability requires specialised expertise. These children require regional assessment (para. 13.3). It is unlikely that the number of children requiring such referral will justify the setting up of 'regional' assessment facilities outside the four Scottish paediatric teaching centres. We recommend that children who are assessed at these regional centres should normally be referred back to the district assessment team, so that the district assessment team may accept responsibility for the management and continuing review of the child in conjunction with his general practitioner. These regional centres should also be concerned with the professional education of the various disciplines involved in the care of handicapped children.

Relationships with education authorities

13.10 The assessment framework which we propose is intended to serve the needs of education authorities as well as health boards. The relationship of the education authority with the team (both at local and district level) needs to be considered. Where the findings of the assessment team may have a bearing on the placement or educational management of a child, further action in that field must lie with the school authority or the education department. Referral of a child to a school doctor and educational psychologist for examination for educational ascertainment (referred to in para. 11.5) is clearly a matter for the education authority, which, at its discretion, may elect to operate within the assessment framework which we propose or to make other arrangements. We recommend that education authorities should be encouraged to use the assessment system which we propose in this report. We also recommend that any proposals made by an assessment team which may affect the placement or educational management of a child should be fed back to the appropriate education authority so that it may take whatever action is necessary.

13.11 We are aware that, in some parts of Scotland, there are groups of professionals having special expertise in particular handicaps who have for some time operated as Special Education Panels. The duty of these Panels is to consider the cases of children who have been subject to the statutory examinations referred to earlier in this report (whether or not these are carried out as part of a process of inter-professional assessment) and to formulate recommendations on the particular requirements of such children for special educational management. The Special Education Panel has a significant role in the process of reaching such decisions and for that reason we identify it in the flow diagram, and show it as linked with both the school assessment team and district assessment team.

13.12 We recognise that any recommendation coming from a multi-disciplinary assessment team which relates to educational management must be translated by the education authority into specific proposals for action. Nevertheless we would be very concerned if there were to be a duplication of assessment procedures to meet the requirements of the Special Education Panels separately from those of the school health service. We recommend that in any areas in which Special Education Panels already exist, every effort should be made to eliminate duplication of assessment by making use of the arrangements which we have proposed in this report. We also recommend that, if our proposals to introduce assessment teams at local and district levels are accepted, there should be evaluation of the need for the continued existence of Special Education Panels.

Chapter 14   District assessment

14.1 We referred in the last chapter to the district assessment team as the second tier in the proposed assessment scheme and to its relationship with both local and 'regional' assessment. We now discuss the functions and membership of the district assessment team and how it relates to the services responsible for the health and welfare of handicapped children.

14.2 The basic functions of the district assessment team which we propose are substantially in line with those suggested for the 'district handicap team' in Chapter 14 of the Court Report. These functions of the district assessment team are also similar to those proposed in Chapter 4 of the Warnock Report in relation to assessment for purposes of educational management. These duties relate primarily to the process of identifying and meeting the needs of individual children who suffer from relatively complex handicap and, in addition, to a general oversight of the services for handicapped children within the area for which the team is responsible. This supervision would extend to children whose initial assessment was carried out by a team from another district. The functions of the team include the provision of support and advice both to parents and also to professional workers caring for individual children. In some parts of Scotland, multi-disciplinary teams with a clinical role are already functioning along the lines proposed in the Court Report. We recommend an extension of these existing arrangements so that all health boards will provide a basically uniform assessment structure in their areas sufficiently flexible to permit any variations which are required to suit local circumstances.

Detailed aspects of the district assessment team

14.3 The term 'district assessment team' may suggest a fixed group in which every member would be equally concerned with each child referred to it irrespective of his particular problem. The concept which we have in mind is more flexible. We visualise a team comprising a small core of members who would provide continuity of method and whose skills would be available to all handicapped children living in the locality, whatever might be the nature of their disability, whether it be physical or psychiatric or mental handicap. Other professionals with special expertise, including those involved in the day-to-day care of the child and familiar with his family circumstances, would be co-opted to the team as appropriate. In this report where we refer to the district assessment team we mean the composite team comprising both the 'core' members and also the co-opted members.

14.4 In suggesting that the district assessment team should deal with all kinds of handicap we have not overlooked the proposal made by the Mental Handicap Sub-Committee of the Mental Disorder Programme Planning Group that there should be a separate team to deal with the needs of the mentally handicapped child. We are, however, anxious that our recommendation that district assessment teams be established should not involve any duplication of provision. The establishment of special teams to deal with mental handicap (or any other special handicap) is bound to create unnecessary complications and to expend resources without appreciable benefit to the child. In particular, we do not see how a child could appropriately be directed to a 'specialist' assessment team where there was some initial doubt as to the nature or extent of his particular handicap. In the case of a child suffering from mental handicap associated with another handicap, he might well be subjected to two assessments. In order to eliminate this kind of overlapping and duplication, we recommend that experts in specific handicapping conditions, including mental handicap, should be co-opted to the district assessment team as the need arises.

14.5 As a step towards implementing the proposals which we make for the establishment of the district assessment team, we recommend that health boards should review the provision now available in their areas and should consider how this can be developed or improved so that every child for whom multi-disciplinary assessment may be necessary can be referred for such assessment at the appropriate stage. Administratively, we consider that multi-disciplinary assessment would, in the majority of areas, be organised most effectively at health district level. We recommend, accordingly, that the initial target should be to provide one district assessment team for each health district; this level of provision will not be appropriate in the case of outlying districts in the Highlands and Islands. Further we appreciate that this target may have to be modified in the light of detailed information on the numbers of children who are likely to be referred for initial assessment, and on the workload arising from such assessment and from the necessary periodic progress reviews. In implementing this recommendation health boards will have to take into account variable factors such as the availability of specialist staff and location of professional resources within their area. These factors are likely to differ widely between urban and rural (and particularly remote rural) districts. There may be scope, in some instances, for co-operation between adjacent districts or even adjacent health boards.

14.6 As indicated in paragraph 14.3 above, the district assessment team will be concerned with assessing the needs of children suffering from complex disabilities living within its area. The team will be concerned with the initial assessment of many pre-school children, as well as of children of school age, and it will also be involved with the review of children of a variety of ages up to school leaving age. In paragraphs 14.22–24 below we deal with the position of children living away from home.

14.7 We expect that, after initial evaluation by the 'core' members of the district assessment team (either individually or working together), certain children would by agreement be identified as requiring multi-disciplinary assessment. Assessment on this basis would necessitate that relevant information about the child's physical emotional, intellectual and social development, his relationships within the family, the community and the school, and his family's material circumstances should be brought together and considered as a prerequisite of planning a programme for his care and management by a multi-disciplinary team, and before any recommendations about his educational management were agreed. Any information available from the child's parents will be invaluable to enable the child's total situation and his needs within the family to be understood. The relationship of parents with the district assessment team is considered in paragraphs 14.19–20.

14.8 In certain children behaviour disorder or emotional disturbance may be as great a problem as the associated mental or physical handicap, and in their assessment and management the district assessment team will have available the resources of child psychiatric and mental handicap specialists. As psychiatric services for children and adolescents are currently being considered by the Mental Disorder Programme Planning Group, this report does not pursue this aspect in depth.

14.9 We recommend that the district assessment team should take a continuing interest in selected children whose care warrants its direct supervision, as well as maintaining the supervision of all children who have been assessed by the team as requiring special measures. This would not necessarily call for detailed routine involvement, but the team would have to verify that the child was in fact receiving continuing care and periodic reassessment at the local level. In certain cases, reassessment might be undertaken by the district assessment team itself. The district assessment team may also have an important role in relation to impending school leavers who still require advice with regard to future employment. In selected cases the district assessment team should be prepared to provide such advice even after the child has left school.

14.10 The general functions of the team referred to in paragraph 14.2 will include advising on the management of children suffering from a wide variety of handicap. Professional workers involved in the care of such children, no less than the children's own parents, need advice and support from professionals with specialist knowledge and skills, and we recommend that the district assessment team should be responsible for seeing that advice is made available to such professionals as and when required through known and accepted channels. We envisage that this function will be shared between the 'core' members of the district assessment team and the co-opted members who have the necessary particular expertise and who work in the local situation (eg those associated with the care of children in special schools).

14.11 The district assessment team should assist professionals working in its area by keeping them up to date with information about the range of services available for helping children so that the professionals can in turn give helpful and consistent advice. Once district assessment teams are established, they will provide a valuable resource for the practical training of students. We recommend that strong links should be maintained between the statutory services and workers in voluntary agencies concerned with the care of handicapped children, and the district assessment team should help in this field. The district assessment team might also have a contribution to make in conducting inter-disciplinary seminars and training courses for workers dealing with handicapped children.

Membership of the team

14.12 We referred in paragraph 14.3 to the distinction between 'core' members of the district assessment team, who would be concerned with all children considered by the team, and co-opted members who would supplement the 'core' members and provide special expertise when assessing a child with a difficult problem. The 'core' members would also have a joint responsibility for the wider functions of the district assessment team discussed in paragraphs 14.9–10 above. We recommend that the 'core' members of the district assessment team should be:

a consultant paediatrician with experience in community child health/ educational medicine.

a nurse
an educational psychologist } of appropriate professional experience and
a social worker } seniority in their respective agencies.

This is as indicated in the flow diagram referred to in Chapter 13 and shown at Appendix G.

14.13 We recommend that the consultant paediatrician should be trained in and have experience of developmental medicine and an understanding of the relationship of paediatrics with education. He must have knowledge of the disorders which are likely to interfere with a child's capacity to learn and of the special needs of handicapped children at school and in the home. In addition to carrying out general paediatric examinations he would have to assess the child's neurological, visual and auditory functions and motor ability. He would have to be able to carry out a preliminary psychiatric screening of any child referred for assessment by the team. The nurse should normally be a registered nurse with experience of handicapped children. The psychologist should be an educational, rather than a clinical, psychologist because it seems desirable, if not essential, to have a representative of the education authority in the district assessment team who is able to command resources and provide a link at the appropriate level with wider expertise. The same kind of considerations apply to the appointment of the social work member.

14.14 It would be inappropriate to list all the professionals who might be co-opted as members of the district assessment team. The list included in the flow diagram gives an indication of some of the main possibilities, and this list is used in our study of the accommodation required by the district assessment team (*see* para. 15.12). While normally only a few co-opted members will be involved at one time, there are bound to be cases of complex or multiple handicap in which more will be necessary. We have included the clinical psychologist as a co-opted rather than a 'core' member of the district assessment team because the educational psychologist representing the education department will act as a 'core' member of the team.

14.15 Without a proper evaluation of workloads it is not possible to say whether there will be sufficient work to occupy the 'core' members of the district assessment team in a full-time capacity. The situation will vary from district to district. Where the employment of full-time 'core' members is not justified, we recommend that the greater part of the working time of such members should be employed in this role. In practice we believe that at least one half of the working time of the 'core' members of the district assessment team will have to be devoted to the work of the team.

14.16 We recommend that the district assessment team should have the services of an administrator who will be responsible for preparing data for consideration by the team, and for arranging meetings and recording decisions. His main task will be to arrange, with appropriate guidance from the 'core' team, for the assessment of children referred to the district assessment team and for review as appropriate of children who have already been assessed. This will involve

F

arranging for the co-option of members, the necessary examinations by the team, co-ordinating the reports on the examinations of the child, completing any other appropriate preliminaries, organising the case conference and circulating appropriate reports. We recommend that the administrator should be a full-time appointment; this will be particularly desirable where the 'core' team is not composed of full-time members. The person selected for this role will have to be a trained and experienced administrator, with a good understanding of the inter-disciplinary nature of assessment, of record keeping and of the preparation of statistical returns and with an ability to organise necessary medical examinations, team meetings and conferences.

14.17 Because of the inter-agency composition of the district assessment team, the reconciliation of the responsibilities of its individual members, whether in terms of their professional role or of their relationship with their employing agency, will be an important element in its effective functioning. In normal circumstances the lead in the 'core' team will probably be taken by the consultant paediatrician, but this will not always be the case. We recommend that at the earliest convenient stage in the assessment of a child the members of the district assessment team should agree which of them will assume the 'lead' responsibility. The problem of professional responsibility is a different matter. Each member of the team must carry personal responsibility and must be free in the last resort to form his own professional judgement, even if this does not conform to the final plan of action agreed by the district assessment team. General acceptance of this fundamental principle should, we believe, improve rather than detract from the effective functioning of the district assessment team, and should encourage the established practice of consultation and co-operation and the free exchange of information and proposals amongst professional workers.

14.18 The provision of a caring and teaching component as part of the assessment system will require substantial support from nursing, teaching and social work staff.

Relationship with parents

14.19 We referred in paragraph 14.7 to the role of parents as the providers of care for handicapped children and to the need for a close association between them and the professional workers concerned with the child. In relation to assessment at any level there is a similar need for the closest possible consultation and co-operation. We recommend, therefore, that parents should be informed at a very early stage in any case where a referral for assessment is contemplated. Their agreement should be sought and they should be invited to participate. Such participation, while not necessarily taking the form of actual membership of the team, should involve the parents in discussions with one or more members of the team. As soon as the team has agreed upon its proposals these should be reported to the parents and their views obtained. The parents should be given an opportunity to discuss the proposals and give them all necessary consideration before any action is taken by the district assessment team. We recommend that the parents should have the right to seek a second opinion in the case of assessment as in the case of any professional consultation. This might take the form of a review of the assessment by a team of professional workers, the majority of whom have not been party to the previous proceedings.

14.20 This kind of comparatively informal arrangement for 'appeal' is not appropriate where the procedure for ascertainment of special educational need is involved as mentioned in paragraph 11.5. Where a decision as to the provision of special education is disputed, the Education (Scotland) Acts 1962–69 provide for its reference to the Secretary of State. On the other hand the increasing tendency of the education authority to exercise its powers on an informal basis as noted in paragraph 11.5 is likely to limit substantially the number of appeals.

Reassessment and review

14.21 Whilst the ultimate responsibility for the health of handicapped children who are living at home or attending day centres rests with the general practitioner, as already indicated in paragraph 14.8 above, the district assessment team should continue to supervise the management of all handicapped children who have been assessed by it. We recommend that the district assessment team should make specific arrangements either to carry out reviews itself or to delegate this responsibility in appropriate cases to the school assessment team. The frequency of reviews and the need for a full reassessment will depend on circumstances. We recommend, however, that reviews should be carried out at least once a year. Parents should be advised on all occasions about the proposed arrangements for the review of their child's case. We recommend that parents should have the right to request a review at any time on providing good reason. The district assessment team may, after consultation with the general practitioner and the teacher, authorise at any time the removal of a child's name from the handicap register if it is satisfied that such a step is appropriate.

Children living away from home

14.22 We are particularly concerned that children who are living away from their homes for all or most of the time should be included in the arrangements for assessment and reassessment. In many such cases there may be an inclination to leave children *in situ* without any alteration in the pattern of management or treatment being provided for them, whereas a careful review might suggest some possible beneficial change. As the practice of multi-disciplinary assessment is extended, it will become increasingly necessary to define professional responsibilities within overlapping geographical boundaries. This should include the coverage of children who are away from home, whether they are in hospitals, in residential schools or in care.

14.23 Such arrangements ought to offer a reasonable balance between the need for assessment of the child in the locality in which he normally lives, and the continuing responsibility of the health and other professional workers in the child's home area (including, for example, in the case of a child attending a residential special school, the primary care team in the home area). The child, wherever he has been placed, should receive the full range of health and other services available. It would, therefore, be entirely appropriate that a child should be referred for assessment (whether by a local team or at the district level) outside his home area if the child is resident in some other area for any length of time.

14.24 Formal notification to the child's home area would only be necessary where multi-disciplinary assessment was being undertaken. We recommend that the district assessment team which functions within the child's place of temporary residence should be responsible both for ensuring that reviews are undertaken, and also for informing the local or district assessment team functioning within the child's home area that it is willing to undertake these tasks. The local or district assessment team functioning within the child's home area would be entitled to decline the offer on the basis that the child's need would be met more efficiently by arrangements made in the home area. This is primarily a matter for collaboration between the appropriate officers of the health boards concerned. It is our concern to ensure that the arrangements which we recommend extend to children in all situations, (including those in long-stay hospitals) and to reduce to a minimum the possibility of children slipping 'through the net' or being ignored.

Chapter 15 District assessment team accommodation

15.1 In paragraph 12.5 we have made a recommendation as to the accommodation in schools required by the school assessment team for the examination of children and for consultation. Adequate provision must be made in schools for visiting services on the lines mentioned in paragraph 12.4. The same applies to local teams dealing with the pre-school child whether they are based on health centres or child health clinics. In this chapter we consider the accommodation required by the district assessment team to enable it to function efficiently and to carry out the comprehensive assessment (outlined in Chapter 14) for which it will be responsible.

15.2 Just as the multi-disciplinary assessment teams which we recommend will serve the needs of both health boards and education authorities, so we visualise that one base will serve the requirements of the district assessment team and act as a centre for observation, assessment, management and education of children. The implications of the inter-agency sharing of facilities are discussed in Chapter 16. We exclude involvement of the social work department in the provision of accommodation because separate assessment centres are operated throughout Scotland by social work departments, as described in paragraph 11.10, among other establishments provided in connection with the social welfare of children. Nevertheless it is essential to include a social worker in the district assessment team staffing proposals which we have made in paragraphs 14.12–18.

15.3 In examining the question of accommodation we concentrate on the general type of facilities which a district assessment team serving a reasonably typical urban area might require. For two main reasons there cannot be one exact model for all district assessment centres. Firstly, any pattern of district assessment centre accommodation will need to be sufficiently adaptable to suit the variety of conditions which obtain within different rural areas. Secondly, in urban areas which have broadly similar conditions, different solutions will be necessary in order to take advantage of any existing provision and to meet the realities of site availability and other planning factors. On the accommodation problem we have confined ourselves in this report to the consideration of the main functions and characteristics of a reasonably 'typical' urban district assessment centre, including its possible use by other services which provide for children in the area. Although our report deals principally with purpose-built centres, we have not forgotten the possibility of converting existing buildings, including school accommodation made redundant by the decline in the birth rate. This must remain a local matter for health boards. The suggestions which are made in this report as to the extent and nature of the accommodation required for a district assessment centre should, however, be helpful to health boards in planning any conversion.

15.4 It is important that the expansion of the existing arrangements for the multi-disciplinary assessment of children should not be delayed until new accommodation is provided throughout Scotland. Depending on the speed with which additional resources can be made available in order to provide the staffing of district assessment teams and the physical facilities necessary for the operation of such teams, there will be an interim period in most areas during which teams must be prepared to use accommodation which is not adequate to meet their requirements in the longer term. The conversion of accommodation could, we believe, produce at an early date temporary facilities which would help to bridge this gap. The provision of temporary accommodation is a diffuse subject and raises questions which can only be answered in the local context, so we confine ourselves in this chapter to purpose built accommodation designed to meet the needs of assessment teams for the foreseeable future, regardless of exactly when it may be possible to provide such accommodation.

15.5 We have not been able to make a detailed study of all the present assessment facilities which are available in the main centres in Scotland nor to evaluate their use in the work of multi-disciplinary assessment. The substantial differences between existing centres have, however, impressed on us the need for caution in advocating a single blueprint for new centres.

General requirements

15.6 As a minimum, the base for a district assessment team must provide office accommodation for the 'core' members, the administrator and support staff, facilities for meetings of the team, consultation/interview rooms, and a records office. Accessibility for members of the team who attend meetings on a regular basis and for health specialists and para-medicals and educational and social work representatives will be important. Facilities should be provided in, or in association with, assessment centres for the extended observation of the children who are being assessed. These will include day nursery school accommodation. Because it is highly desirable that the 'core' members should start working together as a team as soon as possible, if necessary a simplified base should be accepted in the initial stages. The efficient examination and assessment of children may require the provision of some residential accommodation and we return to this topic in paragraph 15.11.

15.7 The lack of statistics makes it very difficult to estimate the number of assessment centres which are likely to be required. Subject to this caution and having regard to the content of Chapter 10, we think that the number of multi-disciplinary assessments required in health district will be sufficient to justify the establishment of a purpose built or specially converted district assessment centre (which together we call an 'assessment centre') in most urban health districts. We recommend accordingly that there should normally be an assessment centre in each urban health district. We also recommend that in areas where urban health districts are close to rural health districts (or, in some cases, rural health board areas) the urban assessment centre should provide as far as possible the assessment facilities required by the adjacent rural health district or area. The situation becomes particularly difficult in remote areas such as the Highlands and Islands.

15.8 We now consider three special factors which influence the location and design of an assessment centre, namely, the relationship of the centre to hospital provision, the age-range to be catered for, and the provision of residential assessment accommodation. We recommend that assessment centres should have their own accommodation rather than accommodation located in, and shared with, an existing hospital. The Court Report (para. 14.41) suggests that the district handicap teams which it recommends should be established should be based on a district general hospital in what is termed in the Report as a 'child development centre'. With respect, we much prefer to locate the assessment centre within the community. We accept that hospital paediatric units will have a major part to play in providing the district assessment team with specialist diagnostic services and probably with accommodation for residential and other assessment when this is not available elsewhere. Indeed, easy access to the resources of such units and close collaboration with the professional staff working in them will be essential for the efficient functioning of assessment centres. We are sure, however, that, while assessment centres should be close enough to paediatric units to be able to obtain the full benefit of their services, they should be located having regard to the community services which are dealing with the children concerned. We recommend that assessment centres should, wherever possible, be separate geographically and administratively from, but nevertheless linked with, children's hospitals or paediatric departments of district general hospitals.

15.9 As regards the age range of the children who should be served by an assessment centre, there is a choice between a centre offering a comprehensive service for pre-school children and a centre offering a range of diagnostic and other facilities at which children can be catered for up to school leaving age. The latter could possibly serve a district assessment team which had an even wider remit than that proposed in Chapter 14; for example, it might provide a base for the mental handicap service for all children within the district concerned. This illustrates what may be an important constraint upon the planning of assessment centres, namely the facilities which are required for the comprehensive assessment of pre-school children do not necessarily fit in readily with those required for the continuing assessment and review of older children.

15.10 We have already stated our view that the district assessment team should be responsible for all cases of children with complex handicap which it has assessed. Such statistics as are available suggest that most children requiring assessment will fall within the age range 0–6, that is the pre-school age group. While we accept that it may be difficult to combine under one roof all the facilities required in an 'all ages' assessment centre, we consider that it should be practicable to arrange the use of the accommodation to make this possible. We recommend that assessment centres should be designed to serve the needs of children of all ages.

15.11 So far as residential accommodation is concerned, the degree of provision must be dictated by local circumstances, including the geography of the area served by the assessment centre, its proximity to a paediatric unit (where the necessary accommodation might be provided more economically) and the scale of operation of the centre as a whole. There will be some centres in which residential provision for both children and parents will have to be included. It may be difficult to make this kind of provision where it involves the conversion of existing buildings, but we recommend that where it cannot be provided at the outset, flexible planning should allow for such provision in the later stages of development.

Optimum accommodation

15.12 As we envisage the working of the district assessment team, the model assessment centre will require to provide accommodation for the 'core' members of the team and for administrative and clerical staff. Consulting or treatment rooms, suitably equipped, will also be required for:

Medical specialists	eg paediatricians, orthopaedic and ENT surgeons, ophthalmologists and child psychiatrists.
Therapists	eg speech therapists, physiotherapists and occupational therapists.
Social Workers	
Health Visitors	
Teachers	eg teachers of the deaf.
Psychologists	eg clinical psychologists.

The list is not exhaustive. In the ideal situation, separate accommodation should be provided for each of these professional staff, but where health professionals are likely to consult infrequently, there may be an appropriate sharing of consulting rooms. Case conference facilities will be essential. It might be convenient for the community medicine specialist to have some office accommodation. There should be accommodation for the secure storage of drugs and medical sundries, eg needles and syringes.

15.13 Day nursery and nursery school accommodation should be provided for the observation, management and care of pre-school children and for the associated nursing, teaching and child care staff. Adequate outdoor play space should be provided, and toy library facilities should be available.

15.14 There will have to be day accommodation for parents who, in many instances, will be working in close association with the district assessment team in the assessment and subsequent management of their child.

15.15 At Appendix H there is a list of the main requirements for an urban assessment centre serving a population of about 200,000 (including a child population of all ages of 50,000).

Chapter 16　Co-operation between health boards and local authorities

16.1 In Chapter 11, we stated our view that any acceptable arrangement for the multi-disciplinary assessment of a child would require to satisfy the needs of health boards and of education authorities to enable decisions to be taken on the care and management of children with handicap. In this Chapter we consider some ways in which co-operation between these two agencies might be improved and in paragraph 16.8 the relationship of social work departments with health boards is discussed.

Involvement of joint liaison committees

16.2 The Mitchell Report[23] refers (paras. 4.1, 4.4) to the need for a close working relationship between health boards and local authorities in various fields. The Report recommends that this can best be achieved by establishing joint liaison committees, the function of which will be to plan a joint approach to the problems which have a common interest for both agencies. In paragraph 4.4(1) of the Report it is suggested that the school health service is one of the fields in which this approach might profitably be employed. We recommend that the joint approach proposed in the Mitchell Report should be extended to the arrangements for assessment and management of children with handicap in which the two agencies have a common interest.

16.3 We recommend that a joint liaison committee at health board or other appropriate level should be established as suggested in the Mitchell Report with as its particular concern the arrangements for assessment of children. Such joint liaison committees should undertake the consideration in detail of the scope, composition and functioning of multi-disciplinary teams on the lines of the 'district assessment team' which are discussed in Chapter 14 of this report. The views which we have expressed in Chapter 14 as to the geographical distribution of district assessment teams suggest that some joint liaison committees may have to contemplate the provision of several district assessment teams operating within their areas. Within the larger regional authorities (notably Strathclyde and Lothian), because they contain the main centres of urban population, the number of district assessment teams will certainly be greater than elsewhere. At the other end of the scale, where 'island' health boards and education authorities are involved, the extent to which local arrangements for assessment can approximate to the model which we have suggested are bound to be limited.

16.4 The main need in the assessment field for formal co-operation between health boards and local authorities will be in relation to the establishment of district assessment teams and the provision of the necessary accommodation. It will also be important for a joint decision to be reached regarding the establishment of 'local' assessment teams (described in para. 13.5).

Boundary differences

16.5 The proposals which we have made regarding inter-agency co-operation in the establishment of assessment teams ignore all problems which arise because agency etc boundaries do not coincide whether they are the boundaries of regional authorities and district authorities or of health board areas or districts as the case may be. The Mitchell Report emphasises the difficulty of achieving full co-operation between local authorities and health boards so long as boundaries do not coincide. Difficulties will inevitably arise where assessment teams comprise professionals serving different agencies with territorial responsibilities which do not correspond. These difficulties will be increased where assessment teams operate across the fields of territorial responsibility of the different agencies concerned.

16.6 Where health district and local authority district boundaries do not coincide, the question arises as to which should be the geographical boundary within which the district assessment team is to operate. This is a field in which there is need for discussion. Because the majority of professionals involved in any session of the district assessment team, comprised as we recommend in this report, are likely to be health professionals operating within health board rather than local authority boundaries, we recommend that the district assessment team should normally relate to a health district or to a health board area. Anomalies are bound to arise. For example, the staff of one educational division may have to deal with different assessment teams. On the other hand, where a school catchment area straddles the boundaries of two or more health districts, children may have to be referred to different district assessment teams according to their place of residence. Such problems will call for local solution as recommended in the Mitchell Report, and will involve close inter-agency cooperation.

16.7 It is not within our remit to make any general recommendation about the adjustment of boundaries in order to achieve coincidence between health authority and local authority boundaries. We emphasise, however, that, as long as these boundaries are not coincident, there will be difficulty in achieving full co-operation between health boards and education and social work authorities in assessment work. This will inevitably increase the complexity and cost of any assessment programme.

16.8 In paragraph 16.2 we have recommended that the joint liaison committees should be concerned with the relationship between health boards and local authorities. The 'input' by the local authority should relate not just to education but also to social work. That the social work and education departments of local authorities operate within different administrative boundaries will inevitably increase the difficulties of co-operation at district level. Apart from this special feature the relationship of social work departments with health boards does not raise problems which differ materially from those already discussed in connection with education. Successful collaboration between health boards and social work departments in assessment work will depend on the contribution made by social workers to the assessment procedures and on the service which can be provided to social work departments as a result of the assessment by district assessment teams of children who are in care or subject to continuing social work supervision. In the present circumstances there would seem to be little scope for social work departments participating in the provision or management of assessment centres along the lines discussed in Chapter 15. On the other hand, the efficient working of assessment centres will be dependent upon a positive contribution from social workers.

Sharing of responsibilities

16.9 Regardless of differences in employing agencies, the collaboration of professional workers in the fields of health, education and social work ought to be effective because of their associated interest in the handicapped child. Questions of responsibility for the implementation and supervision of further action should be resolved as part of the decision making stage in the process of assessment. We recommend that joint liaison committees should assist in this procedure by laying down guidelines so that each agency or professional worker, as the case may be, is able to assume the responsibilities appropriate to its or his particular interest in the child. We are opposed to any proposition that the age of a child, or some similar criterion, should be the basis of decision whether he should be the principal responsibility of one agency rather than another as regards the detection, assessment and management of a handicap. There is a real risk of children 'falling through the net', not only as regards the boundaries within which professional workers of different agencies operate, but also as regards the boundaries of the agencies (health, education and social work) themselves. It was because of this risk that we ascribed a wide co-ordinating function to the district assessment team.

16.10 We recommend that the responsibility for the financing of assessment centres should be shared between health boards and local authorities, with each contributing both to initial capital costs and also provision and financing of staff with the appropriate professional skills. Different local circumstances will influence the proportions in which costs of providing the necessary facilities and staff should be shared.

Reference

[23] *Working Party on Relationships between Health Boards and Local Authorities—Report.* Chairman: J. A. M. Mitchell, Scottish Home and Health Department, Edinburgh, HMSO, 1977.

Chapter 17 Resource implications and priorities for change

17.1 We have considered the priorities for the implementation of our recommendations in the light of their resource implications. It is our view that the recommendations relating to school assessment and regional assessment are not likely to increase significantly either revenue or capital costs but that those relating to district assessment will have substantial financial implications. We have therefore examined the resource implications of our recommendation relating to district assessment.

17.2 We have also considered whether as a consequence of the implementation of our recommendations it is likely that there will be changes in the demand falling on other services. It has been suggested, for example, that earlier assessment might reduce demand for forms of residential care with a commensurate saving in cost. We have concluded, however, that there is insufficient evidence on which to determine whether increases or reductions in demand for this or any other service will result from the implementation of our proposals.

17.3 The recommendations for which cost implications have been considered are as follows:

'The initial target should be to provide one district assessment team for each health district; this level of provision will not be appropriate in the case of outlying districts in the Highlands and Islands'. (Para. 14.5.)

'We recommend that the 'core' members of the district assessment team should be a consultant paediatrician, a (registered) nurse, an educational psychologist and a social worker'. (Para. 14.12.)

'In practice we believe that at least one half of the working time of the 'core' members of the district assessment team will have to be devoted to the work of the team'. (Para. 14.15.)

'The district assessment team should have the services of an administrator'. (Para. 14.16.)

'Whenever possible health and education authorities should combine to provide centres in which care, management and education are provided as an integral part of assessment'. (Para. 11.8.)

'There should normally be an "assessment centre" in each urban health district'. (Para. 15.7).

'Assessment centres should have their own accommodation rather than accommodation located in and shared with an existing hospital'. (Para. 15.8.)

17.4 The recommendations for which we have considered the resource implications may be summarised as follows:

At minimum each health district will have a 'core' assessment team (or its equivalent in terms of resources) which will have the services of an administrator and support staff.

Centres with full facilities for assessment, which will include staff for the care, management and education of children with handicap, should be set up where practicable in each urban health district. The cost of these centres should be borne jointly by health boards and local authorities. For non urban health districts, equivalent resources should be deployed in whatever manner is best suited to the geography and population density of the area.

Method of working

17.5 The method of working which we adopted allowed only very approximate costs to be determined. It should be stressed that the costs presented are intended as a general guide sufficient only to allow the order rather than the absolute magnitude of the resource implications of our recommendations to be identified.

17.6 An initial examination of available estimates of the prevalence of disability in children suggested that it was unlikely that such estimates would provide a basis for quantifying the staff implications of the recommendations. Estimates of the prevalence of disability will depend to a large extent on the definitions adopted. Only a small proportion of children with disabilities will require district assessment. At the same time, there are many children who will require assessment in whom handicap will not necessarily be found.

17.7 Estimates of the likely workload falling upon a district have been based on evidence obtained from an examination of the staffing of existing teams carrying out assessment activities similar to those which would be carried out by the district assessment team which we envisage.

17.8 Data on staffing and workload were obtained from two centres in Scotland carrying out assessment on pre-school children. Information was also obtained on two centres in England carrying out assessment at the English area health authority level. We used these data as a general guide for determining staffing levels which seemed appropriate to the recommendations in the report. Our estimates were based on a notional health district of 200,000 population. Where possible we made estimates of the extent to which, in an area with no district assessment facilities at present, staff would be likely to be transferred from related activities to carry out the functions we recommend.

17.9 In the quantification of Part I of this report in relation to health surveillance we suggested that there would be some possibility of redeploying staff released by the decline in the school population projected for the 1980's. We do not consider that such an adjustment would be appropriate for estimating the staffing implications of recommendations relating to assessment of handicap, since it would appear likely that on the basis of present projections any reduction in the size of the pre-school population in the next four or five years will be reversed by 1987. (See Appendix I.)

17.10 We considered the accommodation which would be required to carry out the functions which we have defined for an assessment centre. (See Appendix H.) Where appropriate members estimated the dimensions of this accommodation drawing upon their own experience and upon information obtained from functioning assessment units. A schedule based on these estimates was submitted to professional advisers of the Building Division of the Common Services Agency, who, with the assistance of other Building Division staff, deduced the likely dimensions of the building. Their co-operation in this task must not, however, be interpreted as approval of the schedule. The approximate cost of a building of these dimensions, excluding site and heating plant costs, was then estimated.

Estimates

17.11 Our estimates on the basis of available evidence for the purpose of determining staffing cost implications of creating a 'core' assessment team in a health district having a notional population of 200,000 are as follows:

a. One half of a whole time equivalent consultant paediatrician post and nurse post will in each case be required to cover the 'core' activities of the team.

b. One administrator and two whole time equivalent secretarial posts will be required for each 'core' assessment team.

c. The additional workload falling on physiotherapy and speech therapy staff arising from the 'core' team's activities will require one half of a whole time equivalent post for each professional group.

80

d. One whole time equivalent nursery nurse post will be required to support the activities of the 'core' team.

These estimates are summarised in Table 5

Table 5 Estimated staff required to provide a 'core' team and associated activities in a notional health district of 200,000 population

	Staff required Whole time equivalents
Staff funded by health board	
Consultant Paediatrician*	0.5
Physiotherapist	0.5
Occupational Therapist	0.5
Speech Therapist	0.5
Registered Nurse* (Sister/Health Visitor)	0.5
Nursery Nurse	1.0
Secretaries	2.0
Administrator†	1.0
Staff funded by local authority	
Educational Psychologist*	0.5
Social Worker*	0.5

*'Core' team members.   †One per district.

17.12 Our estimates on the basis of available evidence for the purpose of determining the costs of staffing an assessment centre in a health district having a notional population of 200,000 are as follows:

a. A maximum of 70 children will be accommodated in the centre during any one session and the majority of these children will attend for the greater part of the day. In addition a small number of older children will attend the centre later in the day after most of the younger children have left.

b. The total staffing of such centres will be as shown in Table 6.

17.13 On the basis that costs will be shared between local authorities and the health service, as we recommend, we estimated the additional number of posts which would fall as a charge on the health service if an assessment centre were to be provided in a health district of a notional population of 200,000 which has no existing district assessment facilities. Our estimates are summarised in Table 7.

17.14 Our estimates of the space required for an assessment centre in a notional health district with a population of 200,000 are summarised in Table 8. On the basis that costs will be shared between the health service and local authorities,

G

as we recommend, only one half of the estimated capital cost of each assessment centre will be borne by the health service.

Table 6 Estimated staff required for an assessment centre in a notional health district of 200,000 population

	Staff required Whole time equivalents
Staff funded by health board	
Consultant Paediatrician	0.5
(Senior) Clinical Medical Officer	0.9
Physiotherapist	4.4
Occupational Therapist	3.3
Speech Therapist	2.2
Clinical Psychologist	1.7
Registered Nurses	
Sister/Health Visitor	2.9
Other	4.0
Staff funded jointly by health board and local authority	
Nursery Nurse/Care Assistant	18.2
Secretaries	3.3
Dining Room Assistant	2.2
Cleaning Staff	1.1
Administrator	1.0
Janitor	1.0
Staff funded by local authority	
Educational Psychologist	0.5
Social Worker	1.1
Teachers	7.0

Priorities for implementation

17.15 In our view the creation of a 'core' assessment team represents the absolute minimum of provision which should be available in each health district, and we recommend that implementation of this proposal should proceed as rapidly as possible. In considering the national cost implications of the full implementation of this proposal we have assumed that, with the exception of the consultant paediatrician, all of the posts required to carry out 'core' assessment team activities in any district will be additional to current provision. In some districts consultant paediatricians at present in post may already discharge many of the functions of the 'core' team paediatrician. Because it has not proved possible to estimate the extent to which this occurs we have estimated as a range the number of new consultant paediatrician posts required nationally to carry out 'core' team activities.

Table 7   Estimated additional staff falling as a charge on the health service required for an assessment centre in a notional health district of 200,000 population

	Staff required Whole time equivalents
Consultant Paediatrician	0.5
(Senior) Clinical Medical Officer	0.9
Physiotherapist	3.9
Occupational Therapist	2.3
Speech Therapist	1.2
Clinical Psychologist	1.0
Registered Nurses	
Sister/Health Visitor	1.8
Other	2.0
Nursery Nurse/Care Assistant	9.1
Secretaries	1.7
Dining Room Assistants	1.1
Cleaning Staff	0.6
Administrator	0.5
Janitor	0.5

Table 8   Estimated space required and cost of an assessment centre in a notional health district with a population of 200,000

Estimated basic building costs per square metre	£220
Area of centre (square metres)	2,100
Basic building cost of centre = £(2100 × 220)	£462,000
Add 'externals and abnormals' at 30%*	£138,000
Basic minimum cost of centre for 70 children, providing 30 square metres per child	£600,000 (1978/79 Costs)

*Externals and abnormals are costs dependent upon the site and other exceptional conditions and which average around 30% but, under particularly adverse conditions, may reach 50% of building costs.

17.16 The total staff implications of the full implementation of our recommendations for 'core' assessment teams are summarised in Table 9.

17.17 The full implementation of our recommendations for district assessment centres will have very large implications both for staffing levels and capital expenditure. Although we attach the highest priority to the full implementation of our proposals, we do not feel that there is sufficient evidence to suggest the timescale over which implementation should occur. This will depend on a variety of factors which will include the provision of staff training facilities and problems of recruitment.

Table 9 Estimated number of additional posts required nationally to meet the recommendations for a 'core' assessment team in each health district

Consultant Paediatrician	7/13*
Physiotherapist	13
Occupational Therapist	13
Speech Therapist	13
Registered Nurse (Sister/Health Visitor)	13
Nursery Nurse/Other Care Assistant	26
Secretaries	52
Administrator	34†

*Range reflects uncertainty as to the extent to which these functions require additional posts.
†One per district.

17.18 Further, we consider that it would be unrealistic to implement a programme of development as extensive as that proposed in this report without taking every opportunity to subject the programme to evaluation. For this reason we recommend that over the next ten years demonstration projects should be carried out in three health districts. This will permit a full research evaluation to be made and alternative methods of achieving our objectives to be contrasted. Results from such studies could be used to modify, as appropriate, later stages of the programme. Initially, demonstration projects should be carried out both in health districts in which little or no district assessment facilities are currently available and in health districts which already have some district assessment facilities. It should be noted, however, that estimates of the cost of our recommendations for experimental centres are based on the assumption that none of the three areas concerned will have significant existing facilities for assessment.

17.19 In recommending demonstration projects in three districts, we do not wish to imply that equivalent staff and capital resources are not required in all districts in order to fulfil our recommendations. We recognise, however, that only after appropriate demonstration projects have been evaluated will there be sufficient evidence on which to make a proper costing of our proposals and to identify how our objectives may be most effectively achieved.

17.20 The cost of our recommendations on three options for implementation is summarised in Table 10. These options are:

Implement recommendations for assessment centres in three districts and 'core' teams in the remainder. (A)

Implement recommendation for 'core' teams in each district. (B)

Implement recommendation for assessment centres in three districts ('core' assessment team functions would also be provided by the staff in these centres). (C)

In costing these options, we have assumed that our recommendations for school and regional assessment (which in themselves have no cost implication) will be implemented in full.

Table 10   Estimated number of additional posts and capital costs falling as a charge on the health service required to meet the recommendations for district assessment of children with handicap three selected options (1978/79 Costs)

	Option A	Option B	Option C
Recommendation to provide 'core' assessment teams in each district	Implement	Implement	—
Recommendation to provide fully staffed assessment centres on an experimental basis in 3 health districts	Implement	—	Implement
Consultant Paediatrician	7/13†	7/13†	2
(Senior) Clinical Medical Officer	3	—	3
Physiotherapist	18	13	7
Occupational Therapist	21	13	10
Speech Therapist	18	13	7
Clinical Psychologist	5	—	5
Registered Nurse			
Sister/Health Visitor	17	13	5
Staff Nurse	6	—	6
Nursery Nurse/Other Care Assistant	50	26	27
Secretaries	51	52	5
Dining Room Assistants	3	—	3
Cleaning Staff	2	—	2
Administrator	33	34	2
Janitor	2	—	2
Capital Costs (as a charge on health service)	£300,000	—	£300,000

†Range indicates uncertainties about extent to which these functions require additional posts.

Conclusion

17.21 Provided that the recommendations in Part I on health surveillance are implemented in full, our proposals for school and regional assessment will have no significant cost implications. It must be recognised, however, that neither of these services can operate at the optimum in the absence of the district assessment team. Until the district assessment team is established, there are likely to be some additional costs in providing regional assessment because the regional assessment team will be the only point of referral for the school assessment team.

17.22 In Table 10 we have considered three options. Only the implementation of Option A will both meet some of the current needs for improved assessment of handicap and provide a basis from which in the longer term a comprehensive assessment service can be developed. Accordingly, we recommend that the priorities for implementation are:

The immediate introduction of school and regional assessment teams on the lines set out in this report.

The establishment as a matter of urgency of 'core' assessment teams as outlined in this report.

The establishment as soon as possible of experimental assessment centres in three health districts to provide a basis for evaluation of our proposals.

17.23 At Appendix J is a note by the Scottish Office Finance Division (Accountancy Services) on the financial implications of district assessment, based on the additional posts required as estimated in Table 6, and considered under the three options of paragraph 17.20.

Chapter 18   Summary of recommendations

18.1 In this chapter we summarise the recommendations which we made in earlier chapters of this part of our report.

SUMMARY OF RECOMMENDATIONS

Inter-relation of health, education and social work services

18.2 Wherever possible health and education authorities should combine to provide centres in which, particularly in the case of younger children, care, management, education and parent counselling are provided as an integral part of assessment. (Para. 11.8)

18.3 Health professionals should collaborate with social workers in assessing the situation of families with handicapped children, taking into account the needs and demands of the family as well as those of the child. (Para. 11.9)

18.4 Assessment procedures required by the school health service and by the social work service should be monitored to evaluate the contribution of each to the assessment of children with complex but related difficulties. (Para. 11.11)

Facilities in schools

18.5 Education authorities should take steps to ensure that both in special schools, and in those catering for a significant number of handicapped children, there should be adequate accommodation for specialist visiting services over and above the normal requirements of the school doctor and nurse and the school dental service. (Para. 12.4)

18.6 (a) The minimum accommodation for school health staff in all but the smallest schools should be a consultation room for exclusive use by the school doctor and nurse, with space there or elsewhere for storage of school health records unless arrangements have been made for records to be kept in health board premises. (Para. 12.5)

(b) Health boards should be enabled more readily to secure exclusive use of accommodation of the standard which health staff require in both new and existing schools. (Para. 12.5)

18.7 All teachers should have training in the health problems of handicapped children as part of pre-service and in-service courses. (Para. 12.8)

18.8 Health board education units should assume responsibility for the provision of any health or first aid information for teachers for which a need may be identified locally. (Para. 12.10)

18.9 The appointment and duties of auxiliary workers to assist teachers with the special needs of handicapped children should be discussed jointly between health and education authorities. (Para. 12.12)

Special requirements

18.10 Where local procedures for the supply of aids and equipment have not yet been agreed between health boards and local authorities and put into operation, action on this important matter should be taken without delay. (Para. 12.14)

18.11 The provision of medical and nursing staff in holiday camps for mentally and physically handicapped children should be a school health service commitment. (Para. 12.15)

18.12 (a) Education authorities should be asked to consider the need for, and feasibility of, introducing more continuous attendance throughout the year at special schools for severely mentally and physically handicapped children.

(b) Education authorities should be asked to undertake responsibility for working out holiday activity programmes for handicapped children, using school premises as appropriate.

(c) Health boards should provide health cover for these children. (Para. 12.18)

18.13 The provision of transport should be discussed by health boards and local authorities as part of their liaison arrangements. (Para. 12.19)

Keeping handicapped children in view

18.4 Health boards, acting through the appropriate Community Medicine Specialist, should assume responsibility for maintaining, updating and reviewing a register at district level of children with handicap. (Para. 12.21)

18.15 The Scottish Home and Health Department should initiate a review of the scope and function of a handicap register. (Para. 12.23)

Tiers of assessment

18.16 School health personnel, in collaboration with colleagues in other disciplines as appropriate, should act as a school assessment team when they meet to consider the cases of school children with possible handicap; this should extend to children attending schools, playgroups or day nurseries at which the school health service provides health surveillance. (Para. 13.5)

18.17 (a) The 'core' members of the school assessment team should be the school doctor and nurse, a teacher with detailed knowledge of the child and the educational psychologist and social worker who have particular responsibility for the school.

(b) School assessment team meetings should be held on a regular basis. (Para. 13.6)

18.18 (a) The school assessment teams for special schools should have their 'core' membership extended to include professionals with expertise in the particular handicap concerned.

(b) Such teams, in addition to their work in special schools, should be available to visit children with the relevant handicap, who are attending local primary or secondary schools. (Para. 13.7)

18.19 Children assessed at regional centres should normally be referred back to the district assessment team, so that the district assessment team may accept responsibility for the management and continuing review of the child. (Para. 13.9)

Relationships with education authorities

18.20 (a) Education authorities should be encouraged to use the assessment system proposed in this report.

(b) Any proposals made by an assessment team which may affect the placement or educational management of a child should be fed back to the appropriate education authority so that it may take whatever action is necessary. (Para. 13.10)

18.21 (a) In any area in which Special Education Panels already exist, every effort should be made to eliminate duplication of assessment by making use of the arrangements proposed in this Report.

(b) There should be evaluation of the need for the continued existence of Special Education Panels if the proposals to introduce assessment teams at local and district levels are accepted. (Para. 13.12)

District assessment

18.23. Existing arrangements for assessment by multi-disciplinary teams with a clinical role should be extended so that all health boards provide a basically uniform assessment structure sufficiently flexible to permit any variations which are required to suit local circumstances. (Para. 14.2)

Detailed aspects of the team

18.24 The district assessment team should co-opt, as need arises, experts in specific handicapping conditions, including mental handicap, in order to eliminate overlapping with assessment teams dealing with specific handicaps. (Para. 14.4)

18.25 (a) As a step towards the establishment of district assessment teams, health boards should review the provision now available in their areas and consider how this can be developed or improved so that every child, for whom multi-professional assessment may be necessary, can be referred for such assessment at the appropriate stage.

(b) The initial target should be to provide one assessment team for each health district, but this level of provision may not be appropriate in the case of outlying districts. (Para. 14.5)

18.26 The district assessment team should take a continuing direct interest in children whose cases warrant its direct supervision as well as maintaining the supervision of all children who have been assessed by the team as requiring special resources. (Para. 14.9)

18.27 The district assessment team should be responsible for seeing that advice is made available to professional workers involved in the care of children with handicap as and when required through known and accepted channels. (Para. 14.10)

18.28 The district assessment team should help in maintaining links between the statutory services and workers from voluntary agencies concerned with the care of handicapped children. (Para. 14.11)

Membership of the team

18.29 The 'core' members of the district assessment team should be a consultant paediatrician, a nurse, educational psychologist and social worker each with appropriate professional experience and seniority in their respective agencies. (Para. 14.12)

18.30 The consultant paediatrician should be trained in, and have experience of, developmental medicine and he should have an understanding of the relationship of paediatrics with education. (Para. 14.13)

18.31 Where the employment of full-time 'core' members of the district assessment team is not justified, the greater part of the working time of such members should be employed in this role. (Para. 14.15)

18.32 The district assessment team should have the services of a full-time administrator. (Para. 14.16)

18.34 At the earliest convenient stage in the assessment of a child, the members of the district assessment team should agree which of them will assume the lead responsibility. (Para. 14.17)

Relationship with parents

18.35 (a) Parents should be informed at a very early stage in any case where a referral for assessment is contemplated. Their agreement should be sought and they should be invited to participate.

(b) Parents should have the right to seek a second opinion in the case of assessment as in any professional consultation. (Para. 14.19)

Reassessment and review

18.36 (a) All handicapped children should be reviewed at least once a year by the district assessment team.

(b) The district assessment team should make specific arrangements either to carry out reviews itself or to delegate this responsibility to the school assessment team.

(c) Parents should have the right to request a review at any time on providing good reason. (Para. 14.21)

Children living away from home

18.37 The district assessment team which functions within the child's place of temporary residence should be responsible both for ensuring that reviews are undertaken and also for imforming the district assessment team functioning within the child's home area that it is willing to undertake these tasks. (Para. 14.24)

General accommodation requirements

18.38 (a) There should normally be an assessment centre in each urban health district.

(b) In areas where urban health districts are close to rural health districts (or, in some cases, rural health board areas) the urban assessment centre should provide as far as possible the assessment facilities required by the rural health district or area. (Para. 15.7)

18.39 (a) Assessment centres should have their own accommodation rather than accommodation located in, and shared with, an existing hospital.

(b) Assessment centres should, wherever possible, be separate geographically and administratively from, but nevertheless linked with, children's hospitals or paediatric departments of district general hospitals. (Para. 15.8)

18.40 Assessment centres should be designed to serve the needs of children of all ages. (Para. 15.10)

18.41 Flexible planning should allow for the ultimate provision of residential accommodation in those centres where this is desirable even though this cannot be provided in the earlier stages of development. (Para. 15.11)

Involvement of joint liaison committees

18.42 The joint approach by health boards and local authorities proposed in the 'Mitchell Report' should be extended to arrangements for the assessment and management of children with handicap in which the two agencies have a common interest. (Para. 16.2)

18.43 A joint liaison committee at health board or other appropriate level should be established as suggested in the 'Mitchell Report' with as its particular concern the arrangements for assessment of children. (Para. 16.3)

Sharing of responsibilities

18.44 Joint liaison committees should lay down guidelines so that each agency or professional worker as the case may be is able to assume the responsibilities appropriate to its or his particular interest in the child. (Para. 16.9)

18.45 The responsibility for the financing of assessment centres should be shared between health boards and local authorities with each contributing both to initial capital costs and also to the provision and financing of staff with the appropriate professional skills. (Para. 16.10)

Priorities for change

18.46 (a) School and regional assessment teams on the lines set out in this report should be introduced immediately.

   (b) 'Core' assessment teams as outlined in this report should be set up as a matter of urgency.

   (c) Experimental assessment centres should be established as soon as possible in three health districts. (Para. 17.22)

Part III
Staffing in the school health service

Chapter 19   Introduction

19.1 This part of our report deals with aspects of medical, nursing and para-medical staffing. Dental staffing is covered in our separate report dealing with Dental Services.

19.2 In Part I of this report we have made recommendations regarding health surveillance within the educational setting. These recommendations are in keeping with the general concept of the school health service outlined in Chapter 16 of the Brotherston Report[24] which suggests changes in the delivery of service rather than in structure. In the foreword to our report it has been stated that it is with some reluctance that we have, as a matter of convenience, made use of the phrase 'the school health service'. Despite our use of this phrase, it is our fundamental objective that there should be one comprehensive health service for all children from birth until they leave school. In this part of our report we have little alternative but to concentrate on the short term position, and we consider primarily, therefore, the service as it now exists.

Reference

[24]*Towards an Integrated Child Health Service*. A report of a joint Working Party on the integration of medical work. Chairman: Sir John Brotherston, Scottish Home and Health Department, Edinburgh, HMSO, 1973.

Chapter 20 Objectives for school health current constraints

20.1 If a school health service were to be created anew within the educational setting, there is no doubt that such a service would differ significantly from the present one. Many of the differences would depend on the organisation of the child health services as a whole. It seems probable that the continuance of existing constraints must be accepted and hence the staffing structure may need to remain substantially as it is. Nevertheless, clarification of the objectives of the school health service should enable the career structure and training of the health professionals involved to be planned within the existing constraints in order to make these objectives more readily attainable

20.2 We believe that ideally the school health service should be organised as a service dealing with health needs related directly to the process of education. The service should not have to devote as much time as is now the case, particularly in primary schools, to health surveillance, because this should be well advanced before children enter school, the majority of handicaps identified and treatment provided where necessary. The service should be able to take a greater lead in the detection, assessment and management of handicap and other child health problems which come to light after the child has started school. We believe that the recommendations in Parts I and II of this report, which deal with health surveillance and children with handicap, serve these objectives.

20.3 We recognise, of course, that the present school health service links with and to some extent overlaps the services provided by general practitioners and primary care teams. Some possible ways of achieving fuller 'rationalisation' of these services have been studied in the Court Report[25] in relation to child health services in England and Wales, and in the earlier Brotherston Report in relation to Scotland. Although full integration may take some time to achieve, much can be done within the present structure to create a more relevant service, and we endorse pilot projects currently being undertaken in some areas. We recognise that staffing and structure are closely related topics. Change in either is not simply a matter of planning from agreed objectives but involves negotiation with and between the professional bodies concerned.

20.4 It is generally accepted that there should be a link between health surveillance of the pre-school child and the service provided after he has started school. As things are now, pre-school surveillance is for the most part provided by different teams which lack common membership. Children below school age do not have to be presented by their parents for screening, and general practitioners have no duty to undertake regular screening examinations of their patients under age 5. In an integrated service, it should be possible to combine the surveillance now provided in health board clinics for children under age 5 with that provided for school children, bringing the primary care team into a comprehensive pre-school service with a more uniform structure.

20.5 Another important issue is the relationship between the school health service and existing specialist services regarding the assessment and management of children with handicap. In Part II of this report we have emphasised that assessment procedures should be designed to ensure the closest co-operation between, on the one hand, school health doctors and nurses, and, on the other hand, the specialist services and primary care teams. We consider, further, that the school health service should have easy access to specialist expertise and advice, and we have made recommendations which we believe should lead to better links with consultant paediatricians and other specialists. The changes which we have proposed relate to the organisation of the service rather than to the creation of any new grade of practitioner.

20.6 Bearing in mind the constraints on reorganisation of the school health service operating in the short term, we have restricted our staffing proposals in the hope that they will not involve any substantial review of basic issues in relation to child health services. Even without major changes in the structure of the school health service in the short or medium term, there are some changes which may come about by gradual evolution. We have not concerned ourselves in this report with staff numbers. It is not within our remit to consider detailed aspects of grading and terms and conditions of service.

20.7 We regard our field of study in this report as limited to the duties of staff, the various professions and professional grades which the school health service requires, the training and expertise required of professional workers and questions of organisation (including relationships between different professional groups) and accommodation. It is on this limited basis that we examine here certain aspects of medical and nurse staffing, as well as the involvement of the main para-medical professions, in the school health service. There are some changes which might be initiated now, even though their fulfilment may not be achieved for some time.

Reference

[25]*Fit for the Future.* The report of the Committee on Child Health Services. Chairman: Professor S. D. M. Court, London, HMSO, 1976. Cmnd. 6684.

Chapter 21 Medical staffing in the school health service

21.1 Over many years the school health service has suffered from the fact that career opportunities for clinicians have been limited, and senior appointments have been administrative in nature and geared to general public health duties. Before 1974, local authority clinical medical officers were mainly employed in the pre-school and/or school health services, though some undertook work in other fields, such as environmental health or maternity services, sometimes in addition to their child health duties.

Position since reorganisation

21.2 The reorganisation of the Health Service in 1974 was recognised as presenting an opportunity for rationalising the child health service as a whole. The Brotherston report considered options for staffing a school health service within an integrated health service for children. It assumed that clinical medical officers would continue, for some time at least, to provide much of the medical manpower required in the school health service, but that general practitioners and consultant paediatricians would gradually become more involved in school health work and would carry out the work previously undertaken by clinical medical officers. It envisaged that, in the future, general practitioners would be able to devote more attention to preventive child health care, and that some consultant paediatricians would develop a special interest in educational medicine, management of the handicapped child and social paediatrics, and that while retaining a role in the hospital field, they would be closely associated with the community health services.

21.3 Proposals for the development of the child health service in Scotland had been framed prior to the passing of the National Health Service (Scotland) Act 1972, and the views of the professional bodies were soon ascertained. Consideration of what should be done to implement the Brotherston recommendations was deferred when the Court Committee was set up in 1973 to study the child health services in England and Wales. The report of the Court Committee was not published until December 1976. Discussions are being held nationally on the future of clinical medical officers as a professional group, and as to their training.

21.4 Both the 'Brotherston' and 'Court' Reports followed broadly similar lines on medical staffing in the future child health service. Court envisaged the gradual establishment of a new type of general practitioner, whom they called 'a general practitioner paediatrician'. This doctor, who would provide general medical services to children and adults in his practice, would also act as adviser on child health matters to his general practitioner colleagues, and would be properly trained in educational medicine so as to enable him to perform efficiently and acceptably as a school doctor. It was envisaged that there would be a gradual absorption of clinical and senior clinical medical officers into the ranks of general practitioners and consultant paediatricians. A new consultant paediatrician was proposed (the consultant community paediatrician). He would be skilled in developmental, social and educational paediatrics and would carry a special responsibility for supporting the general practitioner paediatrician; a consultant working mainly in the community but still engaged selectively in the traditional consultant hospital setting of ward and out-patient clinic. Both reports saw a valuable role for community medicine specialists responsible for child health services.

21.5 At present, almost all medical work in the school health service is carried out by clinical medical officers and only a few general practitioners act as school doctors. In Scotland only one consultant paediatrician in educational medicine has so far been appointed. Hopes that the reorganised health service would attract highly trained doctors into this field who would help to make the school health service more relevant to today's needs have not yet been realised. Nevertheless there is increasing emphasis on community aspects of paediatrics in under-graduate medical education and post-graduate training. The prolonged uncertainty about the future of clinical medical officers as a group must inevitably have some effect on morale in the service as well as restricting recruitment. We understand that in some areas there is a dearth of clinical medical officers due to uncertainty as to their professional future, and that some health boards appear to have assumed that they would be phased out. Inevitably some younger doctors have in these circumstances moved to other branches of the profession. In some areas of Scotland health boards are finding it difficult to provide even a 'skeleton' service.

Medical staffing in the future school health service

21.6 Much of the success of the school health service in the future will depend on its efficient organisation within a structured framework, which will make possible regular monitoring and evaluation, something largely neglected in the past. To bring this about we propose that, as soon as possible, the organisation of the clinical child health service should be the responsibility of the consultant paeditrician envisaged by 'Court'. We agree with 'Brotherston' and 'Court' on the need for different levels of medical expertise in the future service ranging from consultant paediatricians with training and expertise in developmental medicine and the practice of educational paediatrics to doctors carrying out routine school duties, probably general practitioners and/or clinical medical officers. We also see a place for community doctors with special skills and experience in school health but who, either because of the requirements of the Joint Committee on Higher Medical Training, or because they do not wish to carry out full consultant duties, are unlikely to become consultants. Some present senior clinical medical officers could come into this category.

21.7 The community medicine specialists, who would be expected to work in close collaboration with the consultant paediatrician, will have a major task in discerning the pattern of child health in the area (or district) concerned and assessing what relationship, if any, exists between any identified disease and matters of social disadvantage and other social and cultural factors. He will need to work closely with the clinician, especially the consultant paediatrician, in judging how these health needs are being met, the adequacy of services and the use being made of them. He will then be able to pass on this information so that child health needs can be studied with other specialists and the appropriate resources allocated to this field of work. SHHD Circular HSR(74)C3 dated 29 January, 1974 advised that medical officers employed by local authorities primarily as clinicians 'will be on the staff of the CAMO and their work will normally be co-ordinated by the appropriate specialist in community medicine'. Further guidance was to be issued following consideration of the Brotherston Report. We are concerned that the Department has not yet clarified the position of these doctors. We recommend that clinical medical officers working within the community child health service should be part of the clinical divisions of paediatrics.

21.8 In Part I of this report we have already made proposals for the health surveillance of children in ordinary and special schools and for certain groups of pre-school children; in Part II of this report we have made recommendations for the assessment and management of handicapped children. These proposals indicate the type of medical expertise required for the various activities, and, with the range of possibilities which can be envisaged at present, the likely extent of the work to be done. Our proposal is that clinical medical officers and, in some areas, general practitioners with suitable training should undertake routine health surveillance in ordinary schools and participate in the work of school assessment teams. Greater medical expertise is required for handicapped children in special schools, and consultant paediatricians or senior clinical medical officers should normally be responsible for their general health surveillance, and should participate with other medical specialists in the assessment and continuing management of the children. Special Education Panels will need medical representation and social work departments will need medical advice. We think that senior clinical medical officers could appropriately be given these responsibilities in areas where there is no consultant in educational medicine. District assessment teams will need a large medical input from the consultant paediatrician and other medical specialists, whether serving in the 'core' team or as co-opted members. While we would like to see our recommendations for the changes in the pattern of activities in the school health service implemented as soon as possible, we accept that the reorganisation will have to evolve over many years. We hope that, throughout Scotland, a broadly similar pattern of service will be established but recognise that some flexibility will be necessary in order to take account of local circumstances. We welcome the recent Ministerial statement on the continuing role for clinical medical officers and also the discussions that have begun with the profession on their future career structure, training and terms and conditions of service.

21.9 All doctors engaged in school health work require initial training and refresher courses in both preventive and curative aspects of care. We understand that at the request of Health Departments the Councils for Post-graduate Medical Education are considering the future training needs of all doctors who will be involved in child care work; we expect, however, that it will be some time before their proposals are known. Many more teaching staff will be required in academic departments and throughout the National Health Service and more use will require to be made of teaching skills within the community. Every encouragement should be given to the establishment of local pilot schemes for training, making use of all available teaching opportunities, whether in the hospital or community setting. Much more use will have to be made of teachers from other disciplines, and doctors where appropriate should be able to participate with students in other professions. We believe that it is essential that the status of the school health service should be raised and that this should be undertaken without undue delay. If this objective is to be achieved, there is an immediate need for a recognised qualification for doctors intending to practise full time in the community child health service.

21.10 All recent reports on the development of the child health service have stressed the need for greater involvement of general practitioners in health services for school children. We have no doubt that vocational training schemes with a larger child health content will help to motivate general practitioners to undertake school health duties, as will increased contact with school assessment teams. It may not be easy to involve more general practitioners, given their independent contractor status, to take part in school health duties at set times and in a structured service. Paradoxically in rural areas they may be more willing to take on these commitments, since although practice areas are larger the family doctor is more closely involved in the wider community.

21.11 It is evident that, for the foreseeable future, clinical medical officers will continue to be the medical mainstay of the school health service. It is essential therefore that these doctors should receive appropriate training and that they are accepted and recognised as child health clinicians.

Chapter 22 Nurse staffing

22.1 An assessment of nursing need depends first of all on clear policy guidelines on the provision of a school health service. Details and quantification can only be defined with any accuracy when local situations have been considered. In our deliberations we have had the advantage of the National Nursing and Midwifery Consultative Committee (NNMCC) resource document 'A Review of the objectives of the School Health Service and the Role and Function of the Nursing Team under that Service' (1976), to which we from time to time refer.

22.2 We agree with the statement in the Court Report. 'The role of the nurse in relation to education is of the utmost importance and in the past it has tended to be overlooked and undervalued. The school nurse is required to be the representative of health in the everyday life of the school' (para. 10.13). We believe that the school nurse will have an expanding role in an integrated child health service. Her ability to assess and understand the health needs of children and to communicate with them and their parents is of paramount importance.

22.3 Professional isolation can inhibit the development of the service. The school nurse should be a member of the multi-disciplinary team, working in an environment geared to the total educational development of the child and with strong links with the primary care team. She should therefore establish good working relationships with medical, teaching and para-medical staff and others involved, as well as the children and their parents. We support the Court recommendation (para. 10.10) that each school should have a nominated school nurse, and we believe this to be essential to the development of effective communication.

22.4 Close links with the local primary care team(s) will aid the flow of information, but the school nurse will also benefit from participation in case conferences and in-service educational programmes. The school nurse should be based where she can have access to record systems, clerical assistance and receptionist facilities, such as may be provided in a health centre.

22.5 The introduction of a nationally recognised educational programme for school nurses is fundamental to any improvement in the service and we endorse a recommendation of the NNMCC to this effect.

The school nursing team

22.6 The appropriate size of a school nursing team will depend on how best the health objective for a school can be met, and will vary from a sparsely populated rural area requiring one nurse, to an urban area requiring a team of nurses with varying expertise and skills.

22.7 In rural areas, provided that her workload permits, the triple duty nurse, who combines health visiting, district nursing and midwifery duties, is likely to be the most appropriate person to undertake the duties of the school nurse. She will be known to the children and their families and will, therefore, have an understanding of their total situation. She will be working closely with the general practitioner and school doctor as appropriate. The introduction of auxiliary personnel to undertake some duties might be of advantage if the number of children, or the workload, should warrant such an arrangement.

22.8 The NNMCC review suggested that enrolled nurses with additional training could form the core of the school nursing team until such time as the recommendations of the Committee on Nursing[26] are implemented. Thereafter the school nurse should hold a Certificate of Nursing Practice, with an additional 'module' in school health. We agree with these recommendations.

22.9 We further agree with the NNMCC that the skills of registered nurses should continue to be used in special schools and in schools where there is a concentration of children with special health needs.

22.10 A nominated health visitor should be identified with a particular school or group of schools, and should provide advice and support to the school nurse, particularly in schools where there are children with considerable health needs and with behaviour problems. This health visitor will provide the co-ordinating link with the family health visitor and other members of the primary care team, and, assisted by the health education officer and the school nurse, will help to co-ordinate health education. We anticipate that the health visitor will be a participant in the health counselling team.

Areas of responsibility of the school nurse

22.11 a. Health Surveillance. This includes sight and hearing tests, health and hygiene screening, and detection of early deviation from normal. It has been suggested in Part I of this report, which deals with health surveillance, that the school nurse carry out an annual health interview; she may also need to carry out special health surveillance interviews eg before school camp.

b. School Medical Examinations and Immunisation Sessions, working with the doctor.

c. Counselling and Health Education. The school nurse participates in health education and health counselling. We envisage that she will take part in co-ordinated group health education programmes with the health visitor, school doctor, health education officer and teachers.

d. Advice. The school nurse advises teachers and parents on health matters relating to the children.

e. Specialised Experience. Participation in specialist clinics (eg hearing aid clinics) will enable the school nurse to have a wider understanding of the child with special needs.

f. Control of infection. The school nurse has a contribution to make in education on the control and prevention of spread of infection.

g. First Aid. The school nurse should advise the staff of the school on first aid services and on appropriate referral to GPs or accident and emergency units, and might take part in a training programme for school first aiders. She should not be designated the school first aid officer.

h. Home Visiting. There may be occasions when the school nurse will need to visit the home, either to make contact with the parent or to see parent and child together. This may be to follow up children who have failed to attend a special clinic, or, eg, a child not using his hearing aid. This should be undertaken in consultation with the health visitor.

i. Nurses' Clinics. We believe that in areas of high health need, where children or their parents are less likely to make use of primary care facilities, there may be a case for the school nurse being available in school at a regular period each day during which children can be referred by teachers or can refer themselves.

Management

22.12 For a considerable proportion of the day the school nurse will be working alone or with colleagues from other disciplines. The NNMCC state that one health visitor with a reduced case load should be identified as having responsibility for the functioning of the nursing team within each school, and further that this health visitor should have a family case load which should be adjusted accordingly. We agree with their view that health visitors should act as resource personnel, be the point of referral for professional advice and help, and have the responsibility for linking the school both with the home and with the primary care team. However, with the many commitments which health visitors currently undertake and the increasing demands on their time and expertise, we doubt whether, without a distinct increase in staff numbers, health visitors can accept responsibility for the functioning of the school nursing team and the necessary support, monitoring, and evaluation of its work, even with the reduced case load which is suggested.

22.13 We suggest therefore that consideration should be given to an alternative form of management which we believe is already successfully carried out in some areas, where a nursing officer with a health visiting qualification and school nursing experience has direct responsibility for the school health nursing service in a group of schools. There will be situations which merit the formation of school nursing teams; we recommend that there should be a designated leader in each of these teams, reporting to the nursing officer, and responsible for the day-to-day management of the service in each school. A school nurse working on her own would, of course, be directly responsible to the nursing officer. This would in no way alter the need for close links with family health visitors and with other health visitors who are specifically involved in school health counselling and health education.

Auxiliary personnel

22.14 The NNMCC review recommended that the role of auxiliaries within the school nursing team should be to assist within their capabilities whenever and wherever it is appropriate. We agree with this, and suggest that if they are to be involved in special routine screening procedures they should be given appropriate training to ensure a high level of competence.

22.15 Children respond to staff whom they know and trust, whereas a stranger, however proficient, will take much longer to gain their co-operation. A good example is the eye testing of young children. We believe that wherever possible it is better for the school nursing staff to carry out the full range of activities. Delegating single tasks to unqualified staff is, in any event, unlikely to lead to efficiency or to job satisfaction, if only because of their boring and repetitive nature. We accept, of course, the contribution of qualified staff who may undertake specific tests within a range of other duties, eg orthoptists.

22.16 Routine cleanliness inspection and disinfestation, undertaken in isolation from other screening functions, are, in our view, undesirable. Such discrimination can be degrading to the child and may jeopardise his reception of the health teaching relating to his condition. The aim should be to educate the parents and the children to deal with, and prevent, infestation. In this task the lead should be taken by the school nurse, using a nursing auxiliary as appropriate to augment and endorse her teaching. We accept, however, that where parents default from their responsibilities and where there is a persistent problem of infestation, the nursing auxiliary would be the most appropriate member of the nursing team to undertake inspection and treatment and to encourage prevention.

22.17 We consider that there is a place for nursing auxiliary staff to assist the school nurse, wherever there is the necessary workload and a sufficient range of duties within their level of skill. They would be of particular value in areas of high health need where regular hygiene screenings, treatment and teaching are necessary.

Clerical and administrative support

22.18 The school nurse needs access to clerical support, especially when children are starting school and the associated documentation has to be undertaken. The deployment of clerical and other supporting staff must obviously vary according to local circumstances and should be discussed locally between education authorities and health boards.

Children with special needs

22.19 The nursing needs of handicapped children will be assessed before they are placed in an ordinary school and plans made for their management. The Report[27] 'The Secondary Education of Physically Handicapped Children in Scotland' states 'In the case of disabled children, who apart from toileting problems would appropriately be placed in an ordinary school, consideration should be given to the employment of welfare assistants or auxiliaries to provide the necessary help to enable children to attend ordinary schools.

22.20 Some handicapped children will require support, guidance or nursing techniques from the school nurse. We suggest that in schools where the number of such children does not justify the appointment of a full time school nurse a daily visiting service should be provided if appropriate. Where the duties to be carried out are such that they can be taught to, and undertaken by, an un-qualified person, health boards and education authorities should consider the joint appointment of auxiliary personnel, a portion of whose time would be spent on health duties and who should, in respect of this commitment, be responsible to the school nurse.

Special schools

22.21 The needs of children in special schools are likely to warrant the daily presence of a school nurse. The presence of a full time school nurse may be warranted in some special schools. In other schools a nursing team may be required, the numbers, grades and qualifications of staff being determined by the local situation. The team leader should be a registered nurse who has particular expertise with children and knowledge of children with handicap and who has undertaken a course in educational nursing.

Preparation of school nursing staff

22.22 We consider that a nationally recognised course for school nurses should be established as a matter of urgency and, as stated in para. 22.5, we support the recommendation for a 12-week training course. We also support the NNMCC recommendation for a modified form of training to be undertaken, eg a day-release course of 20 sessions, for those already in post.

22.23 Health visitors who participate in the work of the school health service should also be given the opportunity to update their knowledge of educational medicine and nursing. We suggest that the Council for the Education and Training of Health Visitors may wish to consider the developments in the school health service in relation to their proposed review of the Health Visitor Training Syllabus.

22.24 All staff, including nursing auxiliaries, should receive a continuing programme of in-service education.

References

[26] *Report of the Committee on Nursing*. Chairman: Professor Asa Briggs. London, HMSO, 1972. Cmnd. 5115.

[27] The Secondary Education of Physically Handicapped Children in Scotland. The report of the Committee appointed by the Secretary of State for Scotland. Chairman: P. T. McCann, Edinburgh, HMSO, 1975.

Chapter 23   Para-medical staffing

23.1 We acknowledge the contribution of various para-medical professions to the school health service—eg speech therapists, orthoptists, physiotherapists, occupational therapists and chiropodists. Many of these professionals are in short supply, but it is essential that they should take part in the school health service, whether full time or part time. This school commitment should be recognised as an essential part of the contribution of the para-medical professions to child health services. Co-ordination of para-medical services in schools and hospitals is a prerequisite for the best use of therapists and effective implementation of programmes. We urge the para-medical professions to consider how best this can be achieved.

23.2 We see the functions in the school health service of para-medical workers within the school health service as follows:

Screening: orthoptists and speech therapists must be especially involved.

Assessment: multi-disciplinary assessment teams, involving all or any para-medical staff as required, should be available.

Therapy: specific treatment programmes may involve any one of the para-medical professions, particularly physiotherapists, speech therapists, occupational therapists and chiropodists.

Advice to other professionals and parents, particularly on the prescription and provision of aids and appliances and on their proper use, and also in the implementation of treatment programmes.

The planning and development of services, and the integration of medically orientated treatment with the educational programmes in schools, should involve para-medical workers with other professionals.

23.3 It is generally accepted that there is a shortage of para-medical workers, and priorities for their deployment must therefore be considered. Priority in particular should be given to the following:

the younger age group;

children with difficulties in communication; mentally handicapped children (who are often physically handicapped also); supporting services to special schools, whether day or residential.

Constraints

23.4 There is a general shortfall of staff in the para-medical professions which indicates a case for expanding training facilities at pre-registration and post-registration levels, as resources permit. Both initial training and refresher courses should aim to include shared learning with other disciplines. It is important that such training should stress paediatric aspects of care and that wherever possible teaching should be on a multi-disciplinary basis. There should be opportunities for therapists to specialise in paediatric work. Because these are primarily feminine professions, there is a wastage due to workers giving up their jobs because of family commitments. 'Refresher' courses and 'retainer' schemes, which would facilitate re-entry to active practice when family circumstances free the worker, should be established. Ways of attracting more men into these professions should be considered.

Accommodation

23.5 There is a need for adequate and specific accommodation for para-medical services, and for the provision of clerical and support services in schools and assessment centres.

Chapter 24 Accommodation

24.1 Any consideration of school health staffing must take account of accommodation. Most of the work in which school health staff is engaged must in our view be done in the school if it is to be fully effective. Few schools have rooms adequate for interview, treatment and other purposes, and if this state of affairs is allowed to continue it is bound to detract from improvements in organisation and staffing. As improvements are made in the quality of the school health service and as more children with special needs are placed in ordinary schools (rather than special schools), the lack of proper facilities for health staff in these schools will become more evident and less acceptable.

24.2 The basic need in each school, regardless of size, is for accommodation for the exclusive use of the school doctor and school nurse, suitable for clinical purposes and interview and for routine clerical work and consultation between members of the school health team. In addition, there should be suites for visiting services, specially equipped for dental services and able to cater for a range of para-medical services. We recognise that visiting services cannot normally expect to have exclusive use of such accommodation, and some sharing (eg with visiting educational services) may be necessary in the interests of economy. Indiscriminate sharing for totally unrelated school purposes (eg storage space for musical instruments and other equipment) is quite unacceptable.

24.3 Before the reorganisation of the National Health Service in 1974, the school health service was a local authority provision and dependent on the education authority for its accommodation. Though not an entirely satisfactory arrangement, this had the advantage that accommodation problems could, in theory, be resolved within the local authority.

24.4 Under Section 6 of the NHS (Scotland) Act 1972, the local authority had the duty of affording 'sufficient and suitable facilities' for the medical and dental inspection, supervision and treatment of schoolchildren (and young persons attending junior colleges). Subsequently, however, the duty to provide the school health service has been transferred to the Secretary of State (Section 39,

National Health Service (Scotland) Act, 1978) and delegated by him to health boards, which find themselves, as tenants of the local authority, without the freedom to secure the premises which they require.

24.5 The current guidance on this subject, by the Scottish Home and Health and the Scottish Education Departments respectively, is contained in NHS Circular (GEN) 8 1974, which indicates that education authorities should provide 'adequate accommodation, basic services and general purpose furniture', and in an Educational Building Note (No. 13) of 1975, which gives detailed advice on various arrangements to provide suites for visiting services according to the size and type of school, and suggests other forms of provision, (eg for schools where such suites did not exist). We believe that the quality and extent of provision, particularly in older buildings, varies widely and, in the majority of cases, is totally inadequate.

24.6 There would be little problem if this current guidance were fully implemented, both in school buildings designed since 1973, and in adapting older buildings. Present legislation prevents health boards from providing their own accommodation in schools and, as things stand, they cannot require the education authority to meet their requirements.

24.7 We recommend as follows:

(1) Health boards should make their accommodation needs known to education authorities, and programmes of improvement works in individual schools should be agreed.

(2) Education authorities should more readily make available to the school health service space which, because of the drop in the school population, is no longer required for teaching purposes.

(3) The existing obstacles which prevent health boards from contributing to the cost of bringing accommodation in older schools up to the standard required for the school health service should be removed.

Part IV

Child health records

Chapter 25   Introduction

25.1 In earlier parts of this report we have stressed the importance which we attach to the maintenance and development of child health records. Some of our recommendations have direct implications for record practice and others for the organisation and management of record systems.

25.2 We have confined our deliberations in this part of our report to the objectives which should be served by child health records; to suggest how they should be developed would be a task calling for detailed study by professionals and by those who have to make daily use of records.

Chapter 26 The scope of existing child health records and functions of a child health record system

The scope of existing child health records

26.1 A variety of records is maintained relevant to the health of children, extending from the individual child's record to the collection of other data on the provision and use of the health service. Some of these records provide information for clinical management alone; others relate to the use of health services. Many of the record systems at present in use also play an important part in providing information for planning and management, both locally and nationally, and can be applied to medical epidemiological research.

26.2 We are aware that locally there are many child health records which have excellent features; some of these would correspond with our own recommendations. We do not feel, however, that we could do justice to a comprehensive review of local record systems, and for this reason we have examined only record systems which have been adopted nationally. These are summarised at Appendix K.

The functions of a child health record system

26.3 A child health record system should fulfil several distinct functions, not all of which are adequately met by the existing systems. We see these functions in relation to the child as providing:

A record of clinical information.

A basis for ensuring continuity of care and completeness of screening and health surveillance.

A framework to ensure that treatment and follow-up are carried out as required.

Additionally the system should be designed:

To facilitate the flow of essential information between all those with an interest in the child's health.

115

To provide information for the planning and management of health services locally and nationally.

To facilitate the collection of information for medical epidemiological research.

To evaluate the effectiveness of health surveillance programmes.

Chapter 27   Records and health surveillance

27.1 A recurrent theme throughout our report has been the necessity of ensuring continuity of health care throughout the period of childhood. Our recommendations for health surveillance at school were based on the assumption that a comprehensive pre-school developmental screening programme would be adopted throughout Scotland and that information from this programme would be available to the school health service. We have stressed that it is not appropriate for us to recommend a specific pre-school developmental screening programme. We are, however, convinced that such programmes can only achieve their maximum effectiveness if they are linked to a single record on which information about developmental screening, carried out during the neo-natal period and subsequently by general practitioners, clinic staff, health visitors and paediatricians, is collated, together with other information relevant to the health of the child. An integrated child health record need not necessarily take the form of a single document; integration could be achieved by the collation of several documents.

27.2 We recognise that in the development of an integrated child health record there will be many problems relating not only to questions of management but also to the problems of confidentiality which can arise when records from different sources are combined. However, we consider that the value of an integrated pre-school child health record would justify some investment of resources in eliminating these problems.

27.3 We have examined the neo-natal record (SMR 11) now in use in a number of hospitals in Scotland. Although it would not be appropriate for us to comment on its content, we think this record, or one on similar lines, could provide a useful baseline from which to develop an integrated record. Experience drawn from other record systems—for example local immunisation appointment systems—might complement this approach.

27.4 Our recommendations for health surveillance at school have several implications for records. The school health record will require revision if our recommendations to change the programme of examinations are implemented. Any such revision should not be carried out piecemeal, but as part of a comprehensive review, which, among other things, would examine the question of comparability of recording between schools and health boards. Improvements in the comparability of information are essential if the implementation of selective examination is to be adequately monitored. Any review of the school health record card must also seek to enhance the record as a source of clinical information.

27.5 Ideally, a review of the school health record card should be associated with a review of pre-school records. If an overall review is not possible in the short term, we consider that an interim review of the school health record should be carried out as a matter of urgency.

Chapter 28 Communication between professional staff: long term clinical management: provision of information

Communication between professional staff

28.1 In our report concerned with vulnerable families, and in Parts I and II of this report concerned with surveillance and children with handicap, we have stressed the importance we attach to securing improved communication between professional staff concerned with the health of the child. Although improvement in communication will depend largely on organisational changes, and sometimes on changes in the attitudes of professional staff, changes in the practice of record keeping will also be important.

28.2 The integration of pre-school child health records would do much to facilitate communication by providing comprehensive information on each child, which could be passed from one health professional to another. In general we believe that every person coming into contact with a child professionally should have access to such information as is available and is relevant to the discharge of his duties. We recognise, however, that the nature of the relationship between a doctor and his patient may impose constraints of confidentiality on the dissemination of information about the patient. These constraints may be especially acute where information is sought by education or social work authorities.

Long term clinical management

28.3 A major function of child health record systems must be to ensure the follow-up of children with actual or potential disabilities or handicap. The data collected on the present handicap register are very incomplete. If the function of the handicap register is to be extended to embrace surveillance of handicapped children, as recommended in paragraph 12.22 in Part II of this report, then considerable changes in the method of managing the register will be required. Both an integrated pre-school health record and an improved school health record card would help to secure the improved registration of handicapped children.

Provision of information

28.4 Both the effective management and the long term planning of child health services depend on the availability of comprehensive information relating to the health of the individual child and also to the services used by children. At present information collected nationally relates to the neo-natal period, school entry and school leaving examinations, immunisation and in-patient care. There is also the incomplete information recorded on the handicap register. We consider that as a matter of priority not only should existing information systems be reviewed, but also that the information now collected for planning purposes should be extended to include all aspects of child health, and in particular information relating to pre-school developmental screening.

Chapter 29 Recommendations for the development of child health records

29.1 Throughout our report we have stressed our objective that the health of children should be the responsibility of one comprehensive service; it is our view that every effort should be made to achieve integration of child health record systems.

29.2 We recommend that, as a matter of urgency, a comprehensive review should be undertaken of all child health record systems. We recommend that SHHD should initiate such a review, in which particular attention should be paid to the following:

A review of existing record systems, local and national, with the object of developing a nationally adopted record of pre-school developmental screening.

The feasibility of incorporating such a development screening record into an integrated pre-school record covering all aspects of the child's health.

The establishment of more precise definitions with a view to achieving an improved and more comprehensive, handicap register which can be a basis for surveillance.

The revision of the school health record card to secure comparability between its use for recording of defects and its development for monitoring selective examinations.

Arrangements for the continuing review and updating of records.

Appendices

Appendix A

School Health Service: Children examined, per cent with defects[1] by Health Board, school year ending July 1977

HEALTH BOARD

	Argyll and Clyde	Ayrshire and Arran	Borders	Dumfries and Galloway	Fife[2]	Forth Valley	Grampian	Greater Glasgow	Highland	Lanarkshire	Lothian	Orkney	Shetland	Tayside	Western Isles	SCOTLAND
Entrants: Boys																
No. of Examinations	3,669	3,022	748	988	458	2,113	3,688	7,832	1,597	4,301	4,961	122	251	2,798	283	36,831
% with Defects	53.0	53.6	37.0	54.7	47.4	49.3	45.0	51.4	43.6	55.0	50.3	36.1	29.1	52.3	71.7	50.7
Entrants: Girls																
No. of Examinations	3,562	2,878	713	917	504	2,067	3,688	7,528	1,523	4,134	4,815	127	271	2,614	228	35,569
% with Defects	46.0	49.1	34.2	50.3	36.3	42.1	39.2	47.8	38.5	49.1	45.4	18.1	22.1	43.3	72.4	45.1
Leavers: Boys																
No. of Examinations	3,724	2,995	779	1,043	2,365	2,201	3,528	6,269	1,522	3,758	5,029	129	150	2,881	229	36,602
% with Defects	47.3	40.1	37.5	46.9	40.9	33.9	40.9	43.5	41.6	45.3	36.8	24.0	48.0	35.0	26.6	40.9
Leavers: Girls																
No. of Examinations	3,775	3,036	709	1,073	2,332	2,241	3,377	6,414	1,542	3,795	4,923	114	124	3,105	249	36,809
% with Defects	42.8	37.1	38.4	46.8	44.0	35.2	39.7	39.1	41.6	42.2	35.9	28.1	70.2	34.3	21.3	39.2

[1] 'Defects' are abnormalities recorded at the time of medical examination. The presence of a defect does not necessarily imply a disability in the terms of our report.

[2] Fife entrants number incomplete.

124

Content of questionnaires to parents

Because there are many types of questionnaires already in use, and because we consider that the style of questionnaire to be used is a matter for individual health boards, we make no specific recommendation regarding questionnaires, save that undernoted we have detailed the type of data which it might be appropriate to collect by this means. The list is not exhaustive. Some of the suggested items are more relevant to younger children and some to older children. Some questions may have to be repeated before each examination.

1. *General information*

   School.
   Name, address and date of birth of the pupil.
   Name, address and emergency telephone number of parent or guardian.
   Present or usual occupation of father and mother.
   Name and address of the family doctor.
   The number of children in the family and the place of this child in the family.

2. *Immunisation history*

   Whether immunised against

   Poliomyelitis
   Tuberculosis (BCG)
   Diptheria
   Whooping Cough/Pertussis ⎰ age at immunisation if known.
   Tetanus ⎱ any recent booster immunisation.
   Measles
   German Measles/Rubella
   Other

3. *Personal history of the child*

   (1) Birth weight.

   (2) Infectious illnesses.

> Mumps
> Meningitis
> Measles
> German Measles/Rubella
> Whooping Cough
> Pheumonia
> Bronchitis
> Other

and age of occurrence if known.

   (3) *Other illnesses*

> Frequent sore throats or colds
> A running ear or earache
> Squint
> Asthma
> Hay Fever
> Eczema or other skin condition
> Rheumatic fever
> Fits or convulsions
> Any other serious illness or accident
> Previous hospital or dental treatment
> Current medical treatment
> Conditions requiring specific diets

age of occurrence if known.

   (4) *Conditions in which parental observations are particularly important*

> Left handedness.
> Speech problems.
> Snoring or mouth breathing.
> Sleep disturbance.
> Sight or hearing problems.
> Enuresis, by day or night or both.
> Faecal incontinence or soiling.
> Problems relating to puberty.

   (5) *Behavioural or social difficulties*

> Undue timidity.
> Difficulty in mixing with other children.
> Overactivity.
> Destructiveness.

Aggression.
Undue clumsiness.
Persistent disobedience.
Lack of concentration.
Other.

4. *Family history*
   Asthma.
   Eczema.
   Epilepsy or convulsions.
   Nervous breakdown.
   Haemophilia.
   Bereavements.
   Illness in parents.
   Disability, illness or emotional disorder in brothers and sisters.

5. *Any other point of parental concern*

Appendix C

Method of assessing resource implications

Pages 129–131 illustrate our approach to the quantification of our recommendations.

The flow chart on page 129 shows the activities involved in the recommended programme of surveillance as a series of logical steps, and their interrelations.

The table on pages 130–1 shows, as an example of the activities required and the professional staff to carry them out, those involved in the proposed selective examination in the year before transfer to secondary school.

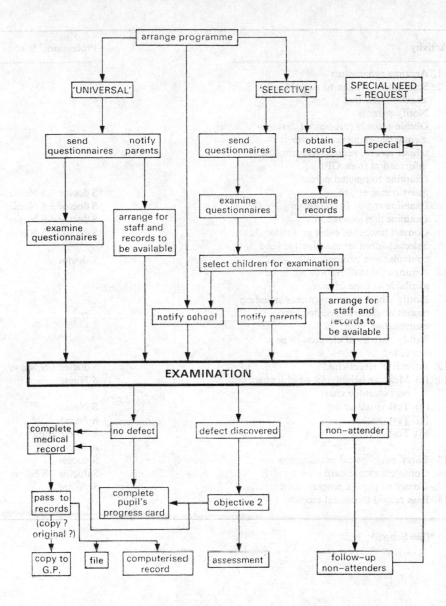

arrange programme

'UNIVERSAL' → send questionnaires / notify parents

'SELECTIVE' → send questionnaires / obtain records

SPECIAL NEED – REQUEST → special

send questionnaires → examine questionnaires

obtain records → examine records

examine questionnaires

arrange for staff and records to be available

select children for examination

notify school

notify parents

arrange for staff and records to be available

EXAMINATION

no defect

defect discovered

non-attender

complete medical record

complete pupil's progress card

objective 2

pass to records (copy? original?)

copy to G.P.

file

computerised record

assessment

follow-up non-attenders

K

129

Activity	Professional Staff
1. Arrange programme	
2. Send questionnaire to parents (not at school leaving)	
3. Notify parents	
4. Obtain records (pre-school developmental screening record, previous school record, request relevant information from GP)	
5. Examine completed parent questionnaires	*S doctor+S Nurse
6. Examine report from teacher	S doctor+S Nurse
7. Examine previous records	S doctor+S Nurse
8. Consult teacher or other professionals	S doctor+S Nurse
9. Select children for examination (and controls: non professional)	S doctor
10. Arrange for staff records etc to be available at time of exam	
11. Notify school of arrangements including names of children selected for examination	
12. Notify parents of children to be examined	
13. Interview parent/child	S doctor+S Nurse
14. (a) Measure height and weight, chart on percentile chart	S Nurse
(b) Test visual acuity	S Nurse
(c) Test urine	S Nurse
(d) Test hearing	S Nurse/audiometrician
15. Carry out physical examination	S doctor
16. Complete record card	S doctor+S Nurse
17. Complete pupil's progress card	S doctor
18. Pass record to central records	

*(S=School)

Contd.

Activity	Professional Staff
19. Copy record to GP	
20. File or computerise central record	
21. Arrange for further action when 'defect' discovered	S doctor
22. Identify non-attenders	
24. Arrange 'special' examination for non-attenders	
23. Arrange and carry out follow-up for persistent non-attenders	S Nurse (home visits)

Projections of expected number of children aged 5, 11 and 16 years in 1981, 1986 and 1991

(using different base year projections by GRO)

	Mid Year Estimate	1973 Base	% Change	1974 Base	% Change	1975 Base	% Change
CHILDREN AGED 5							
1976	83,900	83,482	— 0.50	83,887	— 0.02	84,138	+ 0.28
1981		67,866	−19.11	68,001	−18.95	68,752	−18.05
1986		69,022	−17.73	70,488	−15.99	63,528	−24.28
1991		80,976	— 3.49	89,209	+ 6.33	77,159	— 8.03
CHILDREN AGED 11							
1976	93,700	93,288	— 0.44	93,876	+ 0.19	93,633	— 0.07
1981		86,393	— 7.80	87,508	— 6.61	88,482	— 5.57
1986		69,966	−25.33	70,797	−24.44	72,298	−22.84
1991		71,183	−24.03	73,434	−21.63	66,802	−28.71
ALL CHILDREN AGED 5–14							
1976	897,100	893,000	— 0.46	898.000	+ 0.10	898,100	+ 0.11
1981		778,000	−13.28	784,200	−12.58	792,000	−11.62
1986		703,000	−21.64	714,700	−20.33	686,000	−23.53
1991		771,000	−14.06	824,800	— 8.06	729,600	−18.67
CHILDREN AGED 16							
1976	87,800	87,732	— 0.08	89,275	+ 1.68	87,957	+ 0.18
1981		91,621	+ 4.35	94,356	+ 7.47	92,362	+ 5.20
1986		84,481	— 3.78	87,953	+ 0.17	87,180	— 0.71
1991		68,365	−22.14	71,184	−18.92	70,921	−19.22

Note by the Scottish Office Finance Division (Accountancy Services) on the cost of recommendations: Health surveillance of children at school

1. We have examined Chapter 7 of the report of the Group with a view to placing monetary values on the recommendations made. Eight options are given and against these options the estimated number of new posts for medical and nursing staff that will be required if the proposals are implemented are shown. We cannot comment on the estimated number of posts or on the likely phasing in of these posts over the next eight years.

2. For the purposes of this exercise, we have assumed that any option chosen will be effected in a period of one year. If details of the possible phasing in of the posts are given our figures can be amended, if this is thought to be necessary.

3. In order to be consistent with other exercises carried out recently we have given the estimated costs of the various options at 1975/76 prices. For the purposes of comparison, these costs are given also at the 1978/79 prices. These estimated costs are shown on page 136.

4. As medical and nursing staff costs in the school health service are not separately identified, we could not apply the percentages given in the 'options table' to existing costs. In arriving at our figures, therefore, we have multiplied the additional staff numbers in the table by the average staff costs. The average staff cost has been taken as the mean of the appropriate salary scales. To this we have added an estimated on-cost of 50 % to cover employer's superannuation, national insurance contributions, travelling and other expenses. The on-cost figure which we have used for Higher Clerical Officers (paragraph 5(i) below) is related to the percentage that would be applied with an analogous Civil Service grade.

5. Other assumptions which have been made in arriving at our calculations include:

(i) It has been estimated that every new medical post carries half a Higher Clerical Officer and we have included a provision for this requirement.

133

The cost of the additional Higher Clerical Officers is shown separately and can be deducted if necessary.

(ii) The proposed new nursing posts will not require any new administrative posts to be created, ie any documentation required will be done by nursing or educational staff.

(iii) On the assumption that the visiting medical and nursing staff will spend the main part of their working time in existing premises and will use existing furniture and equipment, no estimate has been made for additional capital expenditure. If it is considered that there is a capital expenditure requirement, we can include this item in our calculations, if details are provided.

Costing of Option Table

1975–76 prices

	Option A	B	C	D	E	F	G	H
	£	£	£	£	£	£	£	£
Cost of nursing staff	175,776	87,888	87,888	29,296 to 73,240	−51,268 to 14,648	−51,268 to 14,648	NIL	−73,240 to NIL
Cost of medical staff	173,840	173,840	NIL	NIL to 86,920	NIL to 86,920	−173,840 to NIL	NIL	−173,840 to NIL
Nos. of supporting clerical staff (HCOs)	10	10	NIL	0 to 5	0 to 5	0 to −10	NIL	0 to −10
Cost of supporting clerical staff	44,250	44,250	NIL	22,125 to 29,296	22,125 to −51,268	−269,358 to −44,250	NIL	−44,250 to NIL
Total cost	393,866	305,978	87,888	182,285 to 29	123,693 to −51	14,648 to −269	NIL	−291,330 to NIL
£'000 say	394	306	88	182 to 182	124 to 124	15 to	NIL	−291 to NIL

135

	A	B	C	D	E	F	G	H
	£	£	£	£	£	£	£	£
Cost of nursing staff	228,624	114,312	114,312	38,104 to 95,260	−66,682 to 19,052	−66,682 to 19,052	NIL	−95,260 to −208,400
Cost of medical staff	208,400	208,400	NIL	104,200	104,200	NIL	NIL	NIL
Nos. of supporting clerical staff (HCOs)	10	10	NIL	0 to 5	0 to 5	0 to −10	NIL	0 to −10
Cost of supporting clerical staff	57,630	57,630	NIL	28,815 to 38,104	28,815 to −66,682	NIL to −332,712	NIL	−57,630 to −361,290
Total cost	494,654	380,342	114,312	228,275	152,067	19,052	NIL	NIL to −361,290
£ 000 say	495	380	114	38 to 228	−67 to 152	−333 to 19	NIL	−361 to NIL

Appendix F

Estimate of prevalence of handicapping conditions (%) derived from various sources

SOURCE	CONDITIONS	AGE GROUP			COMMENT
		0–4 %	5–15 %	0–15 %	
Court[1]	'Physical, motor, visual, hearing and communication handicap, learning disorders' (Sample size = 60,000)	6.0	10.0	8.8	Excludes psychiatric disorders
Bain[2]	'Mental deficiency'	0.3	1.6	1.0	Relates to children screened in a health centre in Livingston New Town in 1971–72. Figures show % requiring continuing medical attention
	'Blind/partial sight'	0.1	0.2	0.1	
	'Deaf/partial hearing'	0.2	0.6	0.5	
	'Cerebral palsy/spina bifida'	0.4	0.3	0.3	
	'Orthopaedic disease/dwarfism'	0.4	0.3	0.3	
	'Epilepsy'	0.3	0.5	0.4	
	'Asthma & Asthma eczema'	1.6	2.2	1.9	
	'Other'*	0.5	0.5	0.5	
	Total excluding enuresis & behaviour disorders	3.6	6.1	5.0	
	'Enuresis'	—	4.4	2.5	
	'Behaviour disorders'	1.8	2.6	2.3	
	Total (Sample size = 3,559)	5.5	13.1	9.8	

*Includes congenital heart disease, cystic fibrosis, coeliac disease, diabetes, neoplasm.

Appendix F—*Contd.*

SOURCE	CONDITIONS	AGE GROUP				COMMENT
		0-4 %	5-15 %	0-15 %		
Miller, *et al.*[3]	'Mental dullness'	5.0				Figures show expected disabilities in 5,000 children entering school in 1952. More than one disability may be present in the same child
	'Severe speech defect'	5.0				
	'Behaviour disorders'	4.0				
	'Growth failure'	5.0				
	'Squint'	5.0				
	'Enuresis'	9.0				
	Other†	3.8				
	(Sample size = 5,000)					
Sheridan & Peckham[4]	'Moderate bilateral hearing loss'		1.2			Covers children aged seven from the National Child Development study sample
	'Severe unilateral hearing loss'		0.4			
	'Marked speech defect'		1.6			
	(Sample size (0-15) = 15,496)					
Birch, *et al*[5]	'Mental subnormality': London		3.6			Aged 5-9
			4.5			,, 10-14
	Middlesex		3.0			,, 5-9
			3.6			,, 10-14
	Salford		2.0			,, 5-9
			2.8			,, 10-14
	England & Wales		2.1			,, 7-14
	Baltimore		1.2			,, 5-9
			4.4			,, 10-14
	Netherlands			2.6		All ages
	Aberdeen		2.7			Aged 8-10

†Includes chronic otorrhoea, chronic respiratory disease, recurrent fits, blindness, deafness, cerebral palsy and other crippling conditions.

138

SOURCE	CONDITIONS		AGE GROUP			COMMENT
			0-4 %	5-15 %	0-15 %	
	'IQ <50'	England & Wales		0.4		Aged 7-14
		Middlesex		0.3		,,　7-14
				0.4		,,　10-14
		Salford			0.4	,,　15-19
		Wessex—Burghs			0.4	,,　15-19
		—Counties			0.4	,,　15-19
		Baltimore		0.3		,,　10-14
		Aberdeen		0.4		,,　8-10
						Reported studies cover the years from the late twenties to 1964
Berger, et al.[6]	'Severe reading retardation':	Isle of Wight		3.85		Compares ten-year-olds in the Isle of Wight in 1965 and an Inner London Burgh in 1970
		Inner London Burgh		9.90		
	'Reading backwardness': (28 months or more backward) (Sample size: Isle of Wight=1,142 Inner London Burgh=1,689)	Isle of Wight		8.3		
		Inner London Burgh		19.0		
Rutter, et al.[7]	'Intellectual and educational backwardness, psychiatric disorders and physical backwardness' (Sample size=2,199)			16.00		Reports on 9-11 year-olds on the Isle of Wight in 1965

References

[1] 'Fit for the Future', Report of the committee on Child Health Services, Chairman Professor S. D. M. Court, HMSO, 1976.

[2] Bain, D. J. G. (1973). 'Health Centre Practice in Livingston New Town', Health Bulletin, XXXI, No. 6.

[3] Miller, F. J. W., et al. (1974). 'The School Years in Newcastle-upon-Tyne 1952–62', Oxford University Press, London.

[4] Sheridan, M. D. and Peckham, C. S. (1973). 'Hearing and Speech at Seven', Special Education, Vol. 62(2).

[5] Birch, H. G., et al. (1970). 'Mental Subnormality in the Community', Williams and Wilkins Co., Baltimore.

[6] Berger, M., Yule, W. and Rutter, M. (1975). 'Attainment and Adjustment in Two Geographical Areas, II—The Prevalence of Specific Reading Retardation', British Journal of Psychiatry, 126, 510–519.

[7] Rutter, M., Tizard, J. and Whitmore, K. (1970). 'Education, Health and Behaviour', Longman, London.

Appendix G

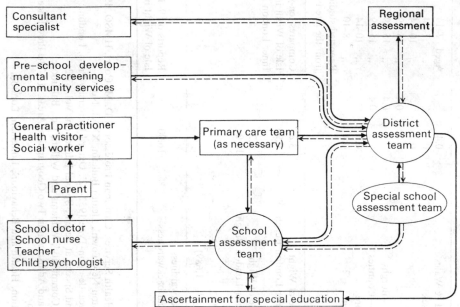

Membership of teams

Primary care team

> *General practitioner*
> *health visitor*
> *district nurse*
> *social worker*

School assessment team

> *Consultant paediatrician in child health*
> *and educational medicine,*
> *experienced child psychologist,*
> *experienced clinical nurse,*
> *experienced social worker.*

District assessment team

Core members

> *School doctor*
> *education psychologist*
> *school nurse*
> *teacher,*
> *social worker*

Other members (co−opted as necessary)

> *Other medical specialists*
> *(e.g. neurologist, child psychiatrist),*
> *specialist psychologist,*
> *specialist social worker,*
> *therapists (e.g. speech therapist)*
> *general practitioner,*
> *school doctor, teacher,*
> *health visitor, school nurse*

List of main accommodation requirements for an urban assessment centre serving a population of about 200,000 (child population of 50,000)

Office for co-ordinator/administrator.
Reception area.
General office for clerical staff.
Records room.
Office for consultant paediatrician and community medicine specialist.
Office for educational psychologist.
Office for social worker.
Office for nurse member of the team.
Staff room.
Conference room.
Waiting room or area.
Parents room/toy library.
2–3 Consulting room, one large with observation bay.
Dental suite.
Physiotherapy room.
Speech therapy room.
Occupational therapy room.
Hearing and vision testing rooms.
Limb fitting and medical appliances accommodation.
4 or 5 Nursery/nursery class rooms.
Outdoor play area.
Toilet and nursing facilities for children.
Dining room and kitchen.
Storage including accommodation for drugs, dressings and medical sundries.
Changing area.
Domestic service room.
Minor laboratory facilities—urine testing etc.
Toilet facilities for parents (adult/handicapped).
Room for mothers to change nappies/breast feed younger siblings.
Toilet for staff.
Loading bay for wheelchairs etc.
Plant room.

Projected child population aged 0–4.

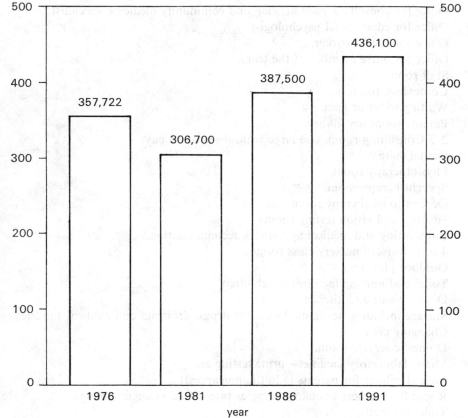

children:
thousands

Source: Projected Home Populations, 1976 based; Registrar General for Scotland

Appendix J

Note by the Scottish Office Finance Division (Accountancy Services) on the cost of recommendations: Children with handicap

As it is considered that the recommendations relating to school and regional assessments are not likely to increase significantly either revenue or capital costs the costing in this appendix is confined to the financial implications of district assessment based on the number of additional posts required as estimated in Table 6 of Chapter 17. A number of assumptions have had to be made in arriving at these figures and the notes following give details of these assumptions.

Table 6

	Option A £'000	Option B £'000	Option C £'000
Consultant Paediatricians	180	180	36
Senior Clinical Medical Officers	40	—	40
Physiotherapists	113	82	44
Occupational Therapists	132	82	63
Speech Therapists	119	86	46
Clinical Psychologists	39	—	39
Sisters/Health Visitors	111	85	33
Staff Nurses	27	—	27
Nursery Nurses/Other Care Assistants	172	90	93
Secretaries	163	166	16
Administrators	200	206	12
Dining Room Assistants	11	—	11
Cleaning Staff/Janitors	15	—	15
	1,322	977	475
Add 2½% to cover contingencies eg travelling expenses, training, etc	33	24	11
	1,355	1,001	486

Explanatory notes

i. The salary/wage scales in force at 1 April, 1978 have been used in arriving at the above figures.

ii. An oncost factor of 50% has been used to cover items such as employers' superannuation National Insurance contributions, administration and accommodation running costs, etc. No element has been included for rent, furniture and equipment as these items will be covered by the capital expenditure.

iii. As the grading and experience of the staff to be employed is uncertain in a number of instances some averaging was necessary.

iv. A range of 7/13 is shown in Table 6 for Options A and B against the number of additional consultant paediatrician posts. In the above calculation a mean figure of 10 was used.

v. The staffing eg educational psychologists, social workers, teachers, which will be funded by local authority is not included in Table 6. As this expenditure will have rate support grant implications (at present 68.5% of reckonable expenditure) it cannot be ignored. It could add approximately £275,000 to Option A, £175,000 to Option B and £125,000 to Option C.

vi. Additional to the cost of the staff tabulated in Table 6 will be professional staff who will be co-opted as members of the district assessment team.

vii. The capital cost of each assessment centre, excluding furniture and equipment, is estimated at £600,000. It has not been possible to obtain estimates for the cost of the furniture and equipment. Although it may be that the capital cost will be shared equally between the health service and local authorities the full amount should be taken into account in assessing the additional charge to the public service.

Appendix K

Summary of principal health records systems with relevance to child health

RECORD	DESCRIPTION	USE FOR CLINICAL MANAGEMENT	USES FOR LOCAL HEALTH SERVICE MANAGEMENT	USES FOR NATIONAL HEALTH SERVICE MANAGEMENT	RESEARCH APPLICATIONS
Individual Case Records ANTENATAL MATERNITY (SMR2)	Record completed on each confinement giving information on mother, pregnancy, labour and limited information on infant	Provides systematic summary for case records. Can be initiated at ante-natal stage	Local systems [but see SMR1 and SMR11] Routine published and unpublished tabulations. Ad hoc analyses	Routine published and unpublished tabulations. Ad hoc analyses	Epidemiological enquiries Date linkage
NEONATAL (SMR11)	Information on condition and care of individual neonates [Incomplete national coverage as yet]	Structured case record for use at bedside. Can be initiated at antenatal stage	Individual Consultant feedback	Routine ad hoc analyses	Epidemiological enquiries
HANDICAP REGISTER SMR7	Record of each congenital or acquired abnormality resulting in handicap in children aged 0–16	NIL	Determination of service needs		Prevalence data [Problems of completeness and definition]
GP RECORDS Forms GP111 EC5B EC6B		Major function			
HOSPITAL INPATIENT STATISTICS—(NON-PSYCHIATRIC NON-OBSTETRIC) (SMR(I))	Record completed for each case discharged from non-psychiatric non obstetric units. Includes patient information, details of clinical management and diagnosis	Provides systematic summary for case record	Routine published and unpublished tabulations. Ad hoc analyses	Routine published and unpublished tabulations. Ad hoc analyses	Epidemiological enquiries, Data linkage
HEALTH VISITOR RECORDS	Many local variations	Individual Child Health Record			
DEVELOPMENTAL SCREENING	Local variants. Not universal	Individual Child Health Record	[but implications for community record]		
SCHOOL HEALTH RECORD SMR10	Record of Defects found at entrance and leaving examination. Use also as school health clinical record	School Health Service use	Monitoring of complete-ness of coverage and defects found	Routine and Ad hoc analyses	
MENTAL HEALTH INPATIENT RECORD SMR4	Record completed on each case admitted to psychiatric or mental handicap unit. Linked record completed on discharge	Provides systematic summary for case records	Routine published and unpublished tabulations. Ad hoc analyses	Routine published and unpublished tabulations. Ad hoc analyses	Data linkage

RECORD	DESCRIPTION	USE FOR CLINICAL MANAGEMENT	USES FOR LOCAL HEALTH SERVICE MANAGEMENT	USES FOR NATIONAL HEALTH SERVICE MANAGEMENT	RESEARCH APPLICATIONS
CANCER REGISTRATION SMR6	Record completed on each case of cancer notified				Epidemiological enquiries. Data linkage
COMMUNITY DENTAL SERVICE TREATMENT RECORD SMR13 [Also EC17 NHS Genera Dental Practitioners Record]	Record of each course of treatment given by the service		Monitoring of use of dental resources individual information for dentists	Routine and ad hoc tabulations	Epidemiological Research
Statistical Returns CLINIC SERVICES & BIRTHS RETURN (ISD(S)7)	(1) Antenatal, postnatal and child health clinic utilisation (sessions and attend- ances) (2) Children referred from clinics to GP or for specialist treatment and advice (3) Live & still births by place of occurrence (4) Deaths in first 28 days by place of birth and birth weight		Workload Information	Workload Information	
COMMUNITY NURSING STATISTICAL RETURN	Return by health board giving: (1) Clinic sessions by type of nursing staff and type of clinic (2) Visits by community nurses by age of patient	NIL	Workload Information	Routine tabulations of Workload Information	—
IMMUNISATION SUMMARY RETURN	Number immunised by age. Based on Form EC72 returned by GP's and clinic returns Local variants. Not universal	NIL	Monitoring of Immunisation status of population	Monitoring of Immunisation status of population	—
IMMUNISATION APPOINTMENT SYSTEMS					
INFECTIOUS DISEASE NOTIFICATIONS	Incidence data on notifiable infectious diseases based on Form EC completed by GPs etc	NIL	Routine tabulations. Data Incomplete	Routine tabulations Data Incomplete	—

Printed in Scotland by Her Majesty's Stationery Office at HMSO Press, Edinburgh
Dd 0630313/3980 K20 8/80 (17078)